Ethics and AIDS

Ethics and AIDS

Compassion and Justice in Global Crisis

Kenneth R. Overberg, S.J.

A SHEED & WARD BOOK
ROWMAN & LITTLEFIELD PUBLISHERS, INC.
Lanham • Boulder • New York • Toronto • Oxford

A SHEED & WARD BOOK
ROWMAN & LITTLEFIELD PUBLISHERS, INC.

Published in the United States of America
by Rowman & Littlefield Publishers, Inc.
A wholly owned subsidiary of The Rowman & Littlefield Publishing Group, Inc.
4501 Forbes Boulevard, Suite 200, Lanham, Maryland 20706
www.rowmanlittlefield.com

PO Box 317
Oxford
OX2 9RU, UK

British Library Cataloguing in Publication Information Available

Library of Congress Cataloging-in-Publication Data
Overberg, Kenneth R.
   Ethics and aids : compassion and justice in global crisis / Kenneth R.
Overberg.
      p.   cm.
   "A Sheed & Ward book."
   Includes bibliographical references and index.
   ISBN-13: 978-0-7425-5012-4 (cloth : alk. paper)
   ISBN-10: 0-7425-5012-5 (cloth : alk. paper)
   ISBN-13: 978-0-7425-5013-1 (pbk. : alk. paper)
   ISBN-10: 0-7425-5013-3 (pbk. : alk. paper)
  1. Medical ethics. 2. Medical ethics—Social aspects.   I. Title.

R724.O94 2006
174.2—dc22   2006016942

Printed in the United States of America

⊗™ The paper used in this publication meets the minimum requirements of
American National Standard for Information Sciences—Permanence of Paper
for Printed Library Materials, ANSI/NISO Z39.48-1992

To the Society of Jesus,
with special thoughts of
Francis Xavier, S.J., John de Brebeuf, S.J.,
the Espinal Community of Cincinnati,
and all those who gather around the banquet table

Contents

Foreword

When HIV/AIDS was first identified in the early 1980s few would have predicted the tremendous loss of life, massive suffering, and global devastation the disease has caused in the last two decades. Though we are still without a cure, there has been major progress in halting the spread and treating the effects of the disease, especially in the United States. Yet, for many in our world, HIV/AIDS continues to destroy the lives of individuals, families, and even entire towns and villages.

HIV/AIDS is a disease which causes disproportionate suffering in those among us who have the least. Poverty exacerbates the devastation as those who are afflicted cannot obtain needed medications or treatments, cannot fight disease due to malnutrition, and cannot prevent transmission due to lack of education and resources. To these members of our human family and to all who suffer, the Church must be a sign of hope.

A distinct feature of HIV/AIDS which sets it apart from the other life-threatening diseases of our time is the stigmatization so many of those diagnosed with the disease feel. Despite large-scale educational efforts, HIV/AIDS continues to be an illness shrouded in fear and mistrust. Paranoia about the spread of the disease on top of hurtful judgments about the way in which one has contracted the virus have alienated persons infected with HIV from their families, friends, employers, and coworkers, leaving them to face the uncertain future of the disease alone and afraid. It is here that we must be a Church of healing and compassion. All of our efforts must communicate a fundamental respect for the integrity of every human person.

The National Catholic AIDS Network is one way in which the Church has responded to the HIV/AIDS crisis. Since its inception in 1989, the organization has worked to coordinate information and resources, provide education and referrals, and to help parishes develop effective programs and services. Many individual parishes and Catholic Charities agencies have made HIV/AIDS a priority in their outreach and ministry efforts. Still, the immense nature of the problem calls for our continued attention and increasing effort if we are ever to bring about a meaningful approach which assures that everyone touched by this disease will experience healing and hope.

Fr. Kenneth Overberg, S.J., has made an exceptional contribution to the dialogue regarding the moral questions which have occurred in the face of the HIV/AIDS pandemic. Utilizing Cardinal Bernardin's Consistent Ethic of Life as a framework, Fr. Overberg searches out the most life-affirming resolutions to issues of life, death, and suffering which cry out for a Gospel response. The issues are far from straightforward, and contemporary debate in the public forum has yielded little consensus. In fact, by contrast, discussion of dilemmas involving abortion, euthanasia, contraception, and needle exchange programs for addicts has created much division both within our own country and among many countries in our world. Those interested in understanding the complexities of these dilemmas will find them concisely articulated here. The tensions which often exist in evaluating these issues from a faith perspective are clearly explained and succinctly analyzed. Fr. Overberg is careful to present the official teaching of the Church, where it exists, and perhaps more significantly, he continually reinforces the respect for human life and human dignity which is at the heart of the Catholic tradition as well as many other faith traditions.

While the bioethical issues are daunting, the societal and worldwide dimensions of the HIV/AIDS pandemic reveal systemic ethical issues involving privacy, confidentiality, justice, and the common good. This book positions those difficult and deeply divisive issues squarely within the same framework of Cardinal Bernardin's Consistent Ethic of Life. It expresses again that our abiding commitment on a social, political, and international sphere ought to be the inherent dignity of human persons and that our consequent decisions must reflect those values which affirm life.

One might not ordinarily expect that a book primarily focused on ethics would include attention to the spiritual dimension of this difficult disease, yet ultimately HIV/AIDS presents both a spiritual crisis and a pastoral challenge. This book offers an appeal to both Scripture and Tradition in an effort to bring a faith perspective on the meaning of suffering and illness to those affected by HIV/AIDS. It will no doubt be of great benefit to both persons who suffer from the disease as well as to their caregivers, family members, parish ministers, and healthcare professionals.

In the 1989 document, "Called to Compassion and Responsibility: A Response to the HIV/AIDS Crisis," the bishops of the United States were explicit in addressing the obligation of the Church with regard to persons with AIDS. "We must keep them present to our consciousness, as individuals and a community, and embrace them with unconditional love. The Gospel demands reverence for life in all circumstances. Compassion—love—toward persons infected with HIV is the only authentic gospel response." The assistance this book offers will go a long way toward making that happen.

Howard J. Hubbard,
Bishop of Albany,
Moderator Bishop
National Catholic
AIDS Network (NCAN)

Acknowledgments

I would like to express my appreciation to the African Jesuit AIDS Network (AJAN) and its director, Michael Czerny, S.J. Inspired by their commitment and challenged by their call to moral theologians to develop sound research, I began this work—and now hope that it can contribute to the response to the AIDS pandemic.

I acknowledge *Presence*, *Spirituality*, and St. Anthony Messenger Press for the use of some of my words and ideas previously published in their publications. I also want to express my gratitude to Dr. Farid Esack, Donna Park, Kathleen A. Parker, Reverend Christopher Ponnet, Barbara Sheehan, S.P., Dr. Patricia Talone, R.S.M., Reverend Robert Vitillo, and my Xavier University students for their insights, corrections, suggestions, and encouragement in making this book a reality.

Thanks to Darleen Frickman, staff assistant for Xavier's theology department, for all her work in preparing the manuscript for publication. Finally, thanks to the Jesuit Community of Xavier University for funding the faculty fellowship for faith and justice that provided time and resources for my work.

Introduction: Confronting Numbness

A growing numbness about HIV/AIDS infects many people in the United States. We fail to recognize that the AIDS epidemic is still getting worse, now spreading rapidly in the world's most populous countries. HIV/AIDS remains a global issue of immense importance, requiring careful reflection, faithful prayer, and committed action.

Our numbness may actually begin in success, the success of the antiretroviral drug therapy that improves significantly the lives of those infected with HIV. As a result, AIDS disappears from the headlines and from our consciousness. Other sources of our numbness may be a weariness with the harsh reality of AIDS around the world or, on the other hand, a lack of awareness of these situations. Perhaps even some prejudice or mistaken judgment that AIDS is an expression of God's wrath causes us to turn away.

To help raise or renew consciousness about this threat to our world, this book summarizes the basics of the AIDS epidemic, presents key themes from the Christian Scriptures and Tradition in light of the Consistent Ethic of Life, analyzes many of the ethical dilemmas raised by the epidemic, and offers suggestions for action. This ethical perspective is the result of decades of dialogue among Roman Catholics and other Christians, building on the strengths of the various traditions. This book offers a Christian view, with special emphasis on Roman Catholic thought; many of its ethical insights, however, can be shared by other faith traditions and by all people who desire to respond to the AIDS pandemic.

Addressing the overwhelming suffering caused by HIV and AIDS is made much more difficult by the presence of widely accepted misconceptions. In wealthy countries both policymakers and ordinary citizens hold such theories as these: (1) HIV/AIDS continues to spread in poor countries because people refuse to change their lifestyles. (2) Antiretroviral treatments are too costly or technically impossible for developing countries. (3) The only option is to concentrate on prevention, not treatment. (4) An AIDS vaccine will soon be available. (5) Ordinary people cannot confront the power of the big pharmaceutical companies. (6) Wealthy countries have nothing to gain by fighting HIV/AIDS in the developing world.[1]

Careful analysis of such statements reveals how far from the truth they are. These false claims lead to passivity and pessimism, stigmatization and numbness. Accurate information, on the other hand, opens up the possibility of hope and committed action.

Because many of us can get trapped by false assumptions, one example can remind us not to jump to conclusions too quickly. It *seems* true that wealthy countries have nothing to gain by helping the developing countries. Serious study shows, however, three long-term gains—in public health, in the economy, in security—from involvement in AIDS work.[2]

First, globalization is leading to increased relations between populations, with greater possibility of the transmission of infectious diseases. Fighting HIV/AIDS now, both in our own country and elsewhere, contributes to the future health of U.S. citizens.

Second, multinational companies are concerned about the effects of HIV/AIDS on both productivity and profits in countries where AIDS is widespread. Studies show that money spent now on treating HIV/AIDS will produce strong economic returns.

Third, in developing countries, AIDS is so pervasive that it attacks the structure of society, creating destabilization and violence within communities and nations. Experience tells us how such violence spills over into the international community. As a result, both the U.S. government and the United Nations have designated the global AIDS epidemic as a threat to national security.

If we move beyond national self-interest, we see that the strongest argument for fighting AIDS is based on morality. We recognize that in our world of many different religions the United Nations' "Universal Declaration of Human Rights" can offer for all a foundation for this moral reflection. From the Christian perspective, our Scriptures and Tradition provide sound guidance for our analysis, choices, and actions.

Staggering suffering and subtly seductive misconceptions present us with many ethical questions. They extend throughout the life cycle and cover the globe. The HIV/AIDS epidemic raises five clusters of moral issues for all who are concerned about human flourishing in our world.

The first cluster is focused on birth, infancy, and childhood. Ought HIV-infected women become pregnant? What methods to prevent HIV transmission ought to be used? Could abortion ever be justified? What is the proper treatment for HIV-infected infants and children? What is society's responsibility for care of AIDS orphans?

A second cluster of ethical questions relates to HIV-infected persons and their relationships. What are their moral responsibilities concerning risky behavior which could infect others? Must they inform current and past sex and drug injecting partners? How do couples decide about their sexual behavior? What about dealings with health care providers: issues of privacy, confidentiality, truth-telling, and using experimental drugs?

A third cluster centers on the end of life. How much pain must be endured? What kinds of life-support treatment are appropriate? Is there a limit to the resources to be used? Is euthanasia or physician-assisted suicide an option?

Society itself faces a fourth cluster of moral dilemmas. Does the common good of society demand testing for HIV, and who will be tested: health-care personnel, those with high-risk behaviors, those who apply for marriage licenses, those convicted of crimes, or everyone? What are societies' responsibilities concerning costs related to HIV/AIDS? Is there a moral obligation concerning educational programs in the light of the growing epidemic? Should programs that promote the use of condoms or needle exchange be supported? What about the effects of prejudice against HIV-infected persons and their families and friends: in housing, parishes, employment, insurance, and medical treatment?

The fifth cluster is perhaps the most challenging, the global structural issues. More accurately, it is one basic question about a cluster of issues: What ought governments do about the economic and social and political structures that contribute to behavior that could spread HIV? Poverty, racism, oppression of women, globalization and the maximization of profits, forced migration, war, and violence of all kinds create the perfect breeding grounds (risky sexual situations and the injection of drugs) for the growth of the HIV/AIDS epidemic. What ought governments and other organizations do to respond, and how can individual persons help?

For many people, especially those in developing countries, addressing these questions remains a great challenge, due to the lack of physical and personal resources. Freedom, for example, is often limited by cultural and economic conditions. Many women may be forced into sex with unfaithful and infected husbands or into prostitution to support their family. Such circumstances have led Lisa Sowle Cahill to conclude: "Personal sin is not the only cause of the spread of HIV/AIDS. In fact, its role pales in comparison to the structures of poverty and gender discrimination that placed most HIV-infected persons at risk."[3]

Ultimately, then, confronting AIDS adequately demands addressing this fifth cluster of global structural issues.

The harsh and horrible reality of global AIDS and this long list of disturbing ethical questions cry out for individual and systemic responses. And so we will turn to the Christian Scriptures and Tradition for the foundation of a vision and for guidance for action. In recent years the development and use of the Consistent Ethic of Life has summarized the richness of the Christian tradition and offered a coherent approach to a wide variety of ethical issues.

Regarding the HIV/AIDS epidemic, these resources help us to appreciate (1) that AIDS is not a punishment sent by God; (2) that Jesus is an example of care and compassion; and (3) that we are called to question and change structures of society that oppress people.

Even as our numbness may be deepening, the deaths and suffering from AIDS continue, particularly in the developing countries. HIV/AIDS may rarely make the headlines these days, but it is devastating the lives of individuals and families, communities and countries. In this context, the Church calls us to live and act as informed citizens and faithful disciples. "The crisis continues, but it can be met with understanding, justice, reason and deep faith."[4]

NOTES

1. Alexander Irwin, Joyce Millen, and Dorothy Fallows, *Global AIDS: Myths and Facts* (Cambridge, Mass.: South End Press, 2003), xviii–xix.

2. Irwin, Millen, and Fallows, *Global AIDS*, 153–67.

3. Lisa Sowle Cahill, "AIDS, Justice, and the Common Good," in *Catholic Ethicists on HIV/AIDS Prevention*, ed. James F. Keenan, S.J. (New York: Continuum, 2002), 291.

4. National Conference of Catholic Bishops, *Called to Compassion and Responsibility: A Response to the HIV/AIDS Crisis* (Washington, D.C.: USCC Office of Publishing Services, 1989), 28.

Chapter One

Basic Facts about HIV/AIDS

We now know many basic facts about AIDS. We also know that we have much to learn as research continues. AIDS (Acquired Immune Deficiency Syndrome) is caused by HIV (Human Immunodeficiency Virus). This virus attacks certain white blood cells called T-cells, eventually destroying the person's immune system. As a result, the HIV-infected individual can suffer from many other infections that a healthy immune system would reject. It is at this stage of HIV infection, with its low T-cell count and various other infections, that the individual is diagnosed with (said to have) AIDS. One of these "opportunistic" infections finally kills the person.

The AIDS virus, HIV, is spread in several ways: sexual contact (including heterosexual and homosexual intercourse), exchange of blood (especially through sharing "dirty" injection equipment for drugs, tattoos, or steroids; "dirty" means that the needle has already been used and contains some blood of an HIV-infected person), and transmission from an HIV-infected mother to her newborn infant during and after delivery. HIV, then, is spread when certain body fluids are transferred from an infected person: in semen, vaginal fluids, blood, breast milk, as well as in the process of birth. HIV can also be transmitted through blood transfusions. While improved screening of blood has almost completely eliminated this danger in the United States, such screening is not available in many countries around the world. HIV is not spread through casual contact: touching or hugging, sneezing or spitting, and using bathroom facilities. We must note that in one sense HIV is relatively hard to spread (only several means are possible), and yet these very means are found in very ordinary activity (sexual intercourse) and in frequent, addictive behavior (intravenous drug use).

Because the means of spreading HIV are few, the means of prevention are evident. Abstinence, faithful marriage between two HIV negative persons, and the use of male or female condoms (also a moral issue to be discussed in chapter 3) would eliminate or reduce the risk of being infected with HIV through sexual contact. Treatment of drug addiction, refusing to share needles, and needle exchange programs (another debated issue) would do the same for those who use intravenous drugs. Treating mothers and newborns with antiretroviral medications, often in combination with elective cesarean section and/or avoidance of breast-feeding, helps to reduce significantly the transmission of HIV from mother to child before, during, and after birth. In situations of poverty, oppression, and inequality, however, such clear means of prevention are often difficult to implement.

Worldwide, the main cause of infection has been heterosexual intercourse, not homosexual activity. Indeed, the late Dr. Jonathan Mann, former director of the World Health Organization's Global Program on AIDS and subsequently of the Harvard School of Public Health, said that if AIDS had been recognized first in Central Africa—as it could have been—then AIDS would be known as a heterosexually transmitted disease which also affects homosexuals. In some countries the epidemic begins with injecting drug use and then spreads through sexual contact. In this context, the words of Pope John Paul II point to a life-and-death issue for individuals and to a profound symbolic challenge for humanity: "The threat of AIDS now confronts our generations with the end of earthly life in a manner which is all the more overwhelming because it is linked, directly or indirectly, to the transmission of life and love."[1] What happens to us as the human family when a fundamental expression of life-giving and love-giving simultaneously becomes death-dealing?

Once infected with HIV, a person (called HIV-positive) is able to infect other persons, even though the infected person shows no signs of the disease. (It should be noted that because of the lack of symptoms, many people do not know that they are HIV-positive. For example, it is estimated that one quarter of the one million people living with

HIV/AIDS in the United States are not aware that they are infected with the virus.)[2] This asymptomatic period, the time from HIV infection to the development of AIDS, can last more than ten years. Just about everyone who is infected with HIV will eventually develop AIDS, but antiretroviral drugs are now able to delay the progression from HIV infection to AIDS in millions of people. The most effective treatment is a combination of drugs called highly active antiretroviral therapy (HAART).

This treatment gives hope of transforming the infection into a chronic disease, that is, an illness that lasts a long time and requires ongoing case management. The antiretroviral medications stop HIV from replicating, gradually reducing the amount of virus in the blood to levels that are not detectable by testing and allowing the immune system to work much better. This therapy is not a cure, as some virus always remains. Although there are problems of side effects and of resistance to some of the drugs, this antiretroviral treatment has greatly improved and extended many persons' lives. For the great percentage of the world's people infected with HIV, however, such treatment is still not available.

The first signs of some kind of a new immunodeficiency condition (later called HIV/AIDS) were described and published in 1981. Since then scientists have done extensive research, initially discovering the virus (HIV) that causes AIDS and eventually developing the combination drug therapies. Many researchers warn us, however, that no quick technological solution for AIDS will be found. HIV is a virus that mutates easily; there are different strains of HIV. All this makes long-term antiretroviral therapy extremely complicated and the development of a vaccine extremely difficult. Realistically, then, we must confront the reality of AIDS and the prospect of living with HIV and AIDS for a long time to come.

The spread of HIV/AIDS continues to increase. Statistics constantly change, but the following numbers give some sense of the magnitude of this global epidemic. By late 2005 an estimated forty million people were living with HIV/AIDS. More than twenty-five million persons had already died, including three million just in 2005. Almost five million people were newly infected with HIV in 2005.[3] The great percentage of these numbers comes from Southern Africa, where in many countries, more than one in five pregnant women are HIV-positive. HIV prevalence among pregnant women in Swaziland reached 43 percent in 2004 (it was

4 percent only twelve years earlier).[4] Even where there are signs of stabilization or even decline of prevalence rates, the reality remains devastating. The stabilization is caused by the high number of new infections now being matched by an equally high number of deaths from AIDS.[5]

In the 2005 report on the AIDS epidemic, the Joint United Nations Programme on HIV and AIDS (UNAIDS) and the World Health Organization stated: "AIDS responses have grown and improved considerably over the past decade. But they still do not match the scale or the pace of a steadily-worsening epidemic. . . . Prevention, treatment, care and impact mitigation goals will have to be pursued simultaneously, not sequentially or in isolation from each other. . . . All this must be done with great urgency."[6]

Urgency, however, continues to be lacking, along with support. The World Health Organization's plan to have three million people in treatment by 2005 "was already [in 2004] collapsing from a lack of money. Donations to the Global Fund to Fight AIDS, Tuberculosis, and Malaria are now about $1.6 billion a year, barely 20 percent of what Secretary General Kofi Annan said was needed when he created the fund in 2001."[7]

The extent of HIV and AIDS is staggering, and the human suffering involved overwhelming. People do not simply waste away from AIDS. Without treatment, often the suffering is intense and prolonged. Many diseases, some of them unfamiliar to most of us, attack the person with AIDS. Later stages may also include explosive diarrhea, lung infections, blindness, and dementia.

If individual human suffering is extreme, so is the cost to society. HIV/AIDS is devastating the developing countries. The greatest percentage of persons with HIV live in these countries. In some countries in Africa, a significant percentage of the population is HIV-infected. A generation of young adults is dying before its time, leaving many children orphaned and leaving the country without new leaders in business and politics. The health-care system, already confronting poverty, civil war, malnutrition, tuberculosis, and malaria, can barely cope with AIDS. As a result, nations are being overwhelmed by the pandemic and face even greater economic and political instability.

In the United States, HIV/AIDS is especially attacking the African-American and Hispanic communities. Almost half of the approximately forty thousand new infections each year are occurring among African-Americans, who make up about 12 percent of the country's population.

For African-American women aged 25–34, AIDS is the leading cause of death.[8]

These communities of color already face a host of problems including racial prejudice, poverty, crime, and drug abuse. Confronting these issues and their relationship to AIDS challenges the nation's political will and its commitment to the common good. The health-care system, under severe economic pressures, faces new demands on its resources as the number of persons with HIV and AIDS increases.

Such sobering global and national statistics have led AIDS researchers to conclude that wherever HIV enters a population, it always moves to those peoples who are already experiencing poverty, oppression, alienation, and marginalization. Acknowledging this reality, Paul Farmer, M.D., has written that "entrenched poverty, economic inequality, racial discrimination, the subordination of women, and other forms of structural injustice contribute overwhelmingly to the spread of HIV infection."[9] With haunting words he also stated that HIV/AIDS has a "preferential option for the poor."[10]

NOTES

1. Pope John Paul II, "A Church Responding to the Sick and the Poor," *Origins* 20, no. 15 (20 September 1990): 244.

2. UNAIDS and the World Health Organization, "AIDS Epidemic Update," *UNAIDS*, www.unaids.org/Epi2005/doc/EPIupdate2005_pdf_en/epi-update2005_en.pdf 66 (accessed 19 December 2005).

3. UNAIDS, "Epidemic Update," 2.

4. UNAIDS, "Epidemic Update," 22.

5. UNAIDS, "Epidemic Update," 17.

6. UNAIDS, "Epidemic Update," 5.

7. Donald G. McNeil, Jr., "Plan to Battle AIDS Worldwide Is Falling Short," *New York Times*, 28 March 2004, 1. By June 2005, one million people had been enrolled in treatment.

8. UNAIDS, "Epidemic Update," 67.

9. Paul Farmer, "Introduction," in *Global AIDS: Myths and Facts*, Alexander Irwin, Joyce Millen, and Dorothy Fallows (Cambridge, Mass.: South End Press, 2003), xx.

10. Paul Farmer, M.D., and David Walton, "Revealing and Critiquing Inequities," in *Catholic Ethicists on HIV/AIDS Prevention*, ed. James F. Keenan, S.J. (New York: Continuum, 2002), 109.

Chapter Two

Ethical Foundations

In order to move beyond the ethics of our society, relativism/ subjectivism (the approach to ethical dilemmas which says that each individual determines the morality of a particular situation), in responding to HIV and AIDS, we must articulate a coherent and comprehensive ethical view. The best of the Christian tradition combines a contemporary understanding of the Scriptures with a reflective view of human life in the world. This chapter, then, presents a moral methodology that takes seriously this "reason informed by faith"[1] approach to Christian ethics, including Scriptural foundations and philosophical insights. The Consistent Ethic of Life pulls together many aspects of past and present wisdom, offering a challenging lens for considering the many ethical dilemmas embedded in the AIDS pandemic.

MAKING MORAL DECISIONS

Some years ago, Christian ethicist James Gustafson suggested that Protestants and Roman Catholics could greatly enhance their ethical systems—and move much closer to each other—by incorporating the strengths of the other group's views.[2] For Catholics, this meant placing Scripture at the very center of ethics and developing a greater sense of historical consciousness; for Protestants, paying attention to philosophical and theological foundations, including a greater appreciation of our shared humanity.

In a brief attempt to provide the foundations of an adequate ethics, the first section of this chapter builds on Gustafson's suggestions and focuses on the WHY, WHAT, and HOW of making moral decisions.

Why

The question of WHY emerges in our experience in a number of ways. At times we may feel overwhelmed by global issues like starvation, AIDS, or the slaughter of innocent people, and so we ask: "Why bother? One person cannot make a difference." Other times, the issue is very close to home: "Why should I try to deal with my prejudice toward people with HIV?"

Why? We get many mixed messages about the meaning of life and about the importance of our moral decisions. We may not be aware of how profoundly and subtly our morality is shaped by our culture. Even as we try to live according to the Gospel, we are constantly bombarded by TV, movies, and advertising—many of which communicate a different set of values.[3]

Life in a consumer society is judged by the clothes we wear, the cars we drive, the electronic "toys" we possess. Success, pleasure, and power are most important. Looking out for #1—whether the self or one's country—is the basic message, whether presented subtly or not so subtly. This emphasis on the individual and individual rights pervades our contemporary society and naturally influences us. "No one can tell me what's right or wrong."

In this context of conflict of meaning and values, we make our moral decisions. Life leads us to make choices. But what directs those choices? The desire to succeed? The hope for pleasure? The fear of punishment? The desire for integrity? The message of Jesus? The wisdom of the Christian tradition? Or some personally developed compromise?

Why try to make moral decisions? Why reflect on the meaning of ethics? The answers are found in the very meaning and significance of our moral choices. These choices really do make a difference because (1) they shape the person we are becoming; (2) they have a real effect on people and the world; and (3) they embody and express our relationship with God.

What we do is intimately connected with who we are. Our choices and the resulting actions shape our very person. Gradually we develop patterns of acting, traditionally called virtues or vices.[4] We become people of compassion, justice, love—or the opposite. A basic stance toward life, sometimes called a fundamental option, develops in and through our significant moral choices, choices about health, sexuality, business, politics, and all the other dimensions of our lives.

These choices also touch the lives of others. There still are real and concrete effects, whatever our intentions and desires. A frightened and abused pregnant woman feels her only option is to have an abortion. Her choice still has a real impact on the fetus (the fetus dies) and on society (it suffers more violence). An international company makes decisions to maximize profits for shareholders. Its decision still has a real impact on its workers in a developing country and on the environment as well.

As we shape ourselves and impact others, we also nourish or damage our relationship with God. Embedded in our choices and actions about ourselves, others, and the world is our response to God, whether expressed explicitly or only implicitly. Indeed, the very heart of morality is first about God loving us and about us loving God. Morality means relationship with God. Our efforts, of course, are never simply human works, but are concrete expressions of our relationship with God. Our moral life is always lived in the world of grace.[5]

The Christian tradition's understanding of moral decision-making is based on fostering and deepening all aspects of our relationship with God. It acknowledges the value of all persons and the interdependency of the world. It stresses that reality—God, human beings, and the rest of creation, all in relationship together—is the basis of morality. Every moral dilemma presents a small but real slice of this reality, that is, in every situation there exists a kind of objectivity—a givenness—something more than just an individual's sincere intentions or strong feelings. Scripture scholar Marcus Borg points to the "givenness" with these words:

> By "is-ness," I seek to express a difficult but obvious notion: namely, that which "is" independently of the maps that we create with language and systems of ordering. Chief among these creations are *social maps* based on culturally generated distinctions. These maps become the source of identity, creating social differentiation and social boundaries. But all of these maps are artificial constructions imposed upon what "is" and what we "are." Beneath the world we construct with language is "is-ness."[6]

Christian ethics leads us to appreciate this value and interdependence, move beyond ethical relativism by acknowledging this "is-ness,"
and recognize that our moral choices have great significance for ourselves, others, the world—and our relationship with God!

Confronting the WHY of morality, however, presents subtle and profound challenges. The challenge is subtle because all of us are shaped
by our culture, yet we cannot stand outside of our past or present to get
an objective view. Values and commitments may well be rooted more in
political and economic worldviews than in the Gospel—as discussions
about such topics as welfare, abortion, and immigration frequently remind us. The challenge is profound because these roots reach so deeply
in our personal lives, grounding our most significant choices and impacting our relationships with others and with God. Uncovering Borg's
"is-ness" takes time and patience.

We need, then, to ask ourselves hard questions. What are our real loy-
alties? How are we influenced by gender, race, class—and all the discussions around these factors? Can we honestly acknowledge the causes
of the culture of violence and death[7] and our role in those phenomena?
How do the Scriptures guide us toward appreciating and nourishing
life?

What

Even when we admit the utmost importance of our moral decisions, we
still may feel confused by what exactly we should do. Whether in the
headline issues or our ordinary lives, many options are presented as the
right one, even within Christianity itself. For example, we may be faced
with deciding what kind of treatment is morally right for a dying parent. Society tells us everything from euthanasia to keeping the person
alive at all costs. While our religious tradition is quite clear on this matter (only ethically ordinary means must be used), it often gets interpreted in very different ways. What are we to do?

Our search for the WHAT of the moral life really implies a dual
search: at the immediate level, the content of a specific moral choice
(e.g., the kind of treatment for my dying parent); at the foundational
level, the kind of person I wish to become (e.g., one embodying compassion, justice, and love). The search at the first level asks: What ought
I to do? The search at the second level asks: What ought I to be?

We have already noted that our culture gives us many—and conflicting—answers to these questions. Again, we need to recognize how influenced we are by these responses. Because our goal ("to be") will shape our means ("to do"), let's first consider what Christianity says about What I/we ought to be?

The Christian tradition helps us answer the question "What ought I to be?" by returning us to our religious roots, the Scriptures, to discern what authentic human life is. While a number of elements can be included, several essential aspects are the convictions that we are created in God's image, that we are bound together in covenant love, that God has become human in Jesus, that we are called to be disciples, and that we are promised new life. Creation, covenant, incarnation, discipleship, and resurrection: these aspects of Christian life form the basis for understanding what it means to be truly human. Different images of God, special concern for the vulnerable and outcast, a sense of solidarity, experiences of reconciliation, and feelings of hope: all these also enrich our sense of the kind of person we are called to be.[8]

Though absolutely essential, this understanding needs further articulation. Insights from Karl Rahner, S.J., help with this task.[9] Based on his careful study, Rahner concludes that all humans share some basic characteristics. (1) The first is that we are body people, and so we exist in a particular time and place. That we live at the beginning of the twenty-first century influences both the way we think and the issues we confront. (2) The second characteristic is that we are spirit people. We are reflective beings who can reach beyond ourselves in knowledge and love. We experience a sense of transcendence, open to and striving for something more. (3) We are also social beings, built to be in relationship with other people. We are interdependent and so have political, economic, and social responsibilities. (4) At the same time, we are unique. Though we share common human qualities, each of us is an individual. (5) Although we face many limits placed on us by culture and family, we possess a fundamental freedom at the core of our being. This freedom is the capacity to choose whether or not to be truly human. (6) The final characteristic is our capacity to be in relationship with God. Humans are capable of encountering the divine.

Scripture, tradition, contemporary experience, and reflection provide important insights into the meaning of human existence, into who we are meant "to be." We are God's people and disciples of Jesus. Intimacy and trust, compassion and forgiveness, and faithful action and concerns for justice characterize our lives. Each person is recognized as an image of God and so is sacred and special. To be human is to be body and spirit, individual and social. To be human is to possess the awesome capacity to say yes or no to this reality of human existence.

Moral choices are those that promote authentic human existence and the flourishing of all creation. Indeed, we say yes or no to "being" in our actions. The WHAT of moral decision-making, then, is also found in what we choose "to do." Perhaps a brief example here will show the relationship between the "to be" and the "to do" question; that is, how reality (the givenness of our lives and actions) is the basis of morality: if to be human necessarily implies being body people, then we have an obligation to care for our health. Our choices to smoke and drink and eat excessively or exercise too little have detrimental effects on our bodies. The "to do" of abusing our health contradicts our "to be" of being body people.

Besides being expressed in the very private choices of the moral life, the WHAT of moral decision-making is also embedded in a whole range of political, social, and economic decisions and actions (more examples of "to do"). In recent years various liberation theologies and the social teachings of the church have drawn attention to welfare and immigration, sexism and racism, abortion and health care, euthanasia and the death penalty, genocide and trade agreements, and many other urgent issues rooted in human social solidarity. We have already seen hints that HIV and AIDS are connected to many of these issues.

We need to be especially sensitive to this solidarity and interdependence. Social, economic, and political issues in our communities and around the world are religious and moral issues. And they are necessarily our concern. Making the connections between our personal particular topics and these wider issues—justice in the church and in society, for example—will lead us to a richer sense of human flourishing and to a greater sensitivity to the WHAT of moral reasoning.

People of faith have long attempted to discern what actions will truly lead to this flourishing. Religion at its best does not tell us what to do; rather, it provides guidance based on this kind of discernment. Wisdom grows from experience and eventually gets expressed in laws; that is how the Ten Commandments developed, for example.

Christian ethics, then, helps us to remember that both character issues ("to be") and specific actions ("to do") are significant. The recent renewal and rapprochement in Christian ethics challenges us to focus on the "being" and "doing" of Jesus and to evaluate human actions on the basis of the whole person understood in historical context. In the next section, we will return to the example of Jesus and its importance for our response to HIV and AIDS.

How

We have looked at the WHY (intention) and the WHAT (content) of Christian ethics. Our third area is method. HOW do we go about making moral decisions? Most major moral decisions are made by using one of the three following approaches.

Many of us were taught to make moral decisions by following the law. Understand the situation, find the appropriate law, obey. Some authority, whether Jesus or Scripture or pope, decided what was right. Experience, however, has led many of us to realize that sometimes the letter of the law oppresses the spirit or simply cannot deal with the complexity of a particular case.

Our culture gives us very different direction. "If it feels good, do it!" "Each person must decide for himself or herself." Simply by living in our culture, most if not all of us have been deeply influenced by the individualism and emphasis on individual rights. Instead of carefully considering the moral implications of the action itself, this type of thinking, relativism, holds that the individual's sincere intentions alone (or the good consequences) are enough to make the action morally right.

Christian reflection on morality long ago developed a third view, which focuses on the use of discernment. Recent renewal has returned to the heart of this method, although discussion and debate continue about how best to make moral decisions. This third view holds that after careful discernment the individual must decide, but always in the context of the community's wisdom and with an understanding of what is *really* happening—not what one *would like* to happen. There is a certain objectivity to our actions; as was discussed earlier, actions have real meanings and consequences.

Most of our choices contain positive and negative aspects. For example, reading a good book means less time working in the garden; more significantly, saving a life may mean amputating a leg full of gangrene. At the heart of our discernment is the prayerful weighing of these competing values and disvalues. Does saving a life justify cutting off a leg? Most of us would answer a definite yes. Other situations are not so clear, and yet this delicate balancing and discernment has been central to moral decision-making. The goal of this balancing and discernment, of course, is to discover the choice that most fully promotes true human flourishing. Such discernment demands careful consideration of all aspects of the moral dilemma, traditionally named "act, intention, and circumstances."[10] Because we cannot always see clearly, the wisdom of tradition and authority can be especially helpful at this point.

The HOW of moral decision-making is no easy task. For it demands a careful avoiding of extremes, a delicate dealing with deeply embedded patterns, a recognition of the strengths and weaknesses of our own religious tradition. On the one side is relativism, the morality of our culture, a pervasive and powerful force. It is almost impossible to escape its seductive simplicity: "Only you can determine what is the loving thing to do in this specific situation." On the other side is law and obedience, the power of tradition, promising clarity and certainty. For some people, such obedience may be a warm security blanket; for others, this approach may lead to scruples.

We search for virtue somewhere between the extremes. We recognize the proper role of authority and the wisdom of law but also appreciate the uniqueness of each situation and the freedom and responsibility of the mature decision-maker. We try to see clearly the realities of every moral dilemma (not just good intentions), to grow in confidence in discerning a sincere and correct response to such dilemmas, and to live out the decision in peace.

Conscience too plays a central role in this discernment. Conscience is not a little voice or some inner police officer. It is simply the person trying to make sound judgments about moral questions. Our conscience does not suddenly appear, fully formed. No, it needs to be developed— a process traditionally called "the formation of conscience."

In *Principles for a Catholic Morality*, Timothy O'Connell summarizes the tradition and presents a very concise and helpful picture of conscience, describing it as three different dimensions of a person.[11] The first dimension of conscience is *a capacity*: the general sense of value that is characteristic of the human being. We are aware that we should do good and avoid evil. The second dimension of conscience is *a process*: the search to discover the right course of action. This probing into human behavior and the world is the search for truth. If we are honest in our search, then we turn to a variety of wisdom sources: scripture, the Church, physical and human sciences, tradition, and competent professional advice. The third dimension of conscience is *a decision*: the actual, concrete judgment that we make pertaining to an immediate action.

We must follow our conscience but only after doing our best at this search for the truth, the WHY and WHAT of the earlier sections of this chapter. There may appear to be a tension between conscience and truth. That is why O'Connell says that, even though a sincere conscience may safeguard the individual's relationship with God, a sincere conscience also wants to be correct.[12] Here "correct" means that the individual has accurately discerned which action most fully promotes true human flourishing.

Following our conscience and weighing competing values does not mean doing what we feel like doing. It does mean the hard work of discerning what is right and what is wrong. It does mean recognizing the meaning of the mystery of Christ for our lives, appreciating the historical context and social solidarity of our lives, taking seriously the wisdom of tradition and guidance of authority, and acknowledging the complexity of contemporary moral dilemmas and the role of personal responsibility. In short, it means the challenge of mature moral decision-making.

Both rigidity and fear of change and the materialism and relativism of our culture limit and distort the rich resources of Christian ethics. Appreciating the WHY, WHAT, and HOW of a morality rooted in the strengths of various Christian perspectives renews the coherence and adequacy of our ethics and helps us to respond with hope and vision to the ethical dilemmas of our day, including the complex issues of the AIDS pandemic.

BIBLICAL ROOTS

Having described a method for making moral decisions, let's now return to Scripture for a more detailed foundation for a response to the ethical issues that HIV/AIDS raises throughout the life cycle and around the globe.

Two biblical convictions and one condition provide the context for developing a biblical vision of AIDS. The condition is leprosy; the first conviction holds that disease is not a punishment from God; the second conviction proclaims a faith that does justice. Underlying these convictions, of course, is the more foundational belief that all people are created in God's image and called to everlasting life.

Sickness As Punishment

Let's begin with the first conviction. Deeply embedded in some streams of Hebrew thought was the sense that good deeds led to blessing and evil deeds to suffering. If a person were experiencing sickness or other trials, then that person must have sinned in the past. This perspective is grounded in the Deuteronomy tradition and is perfectly expressed by Job's "friends" (see the series of speeches in chapters 3–31). The Book of Job, however, challenges this tradition; Job suffers despite his innocence (Job 31 especially).

Jesus too challenges this belief. In the exquisite scene described in chapter nine of John's Gospel, Jesus heals a blind man. Then threats, excuses, and faith take center stage. Even before the healing, Jesus declares that the man's blindness was not due to his or his parents' sin (John 9:2–5). Neither Job nor Jesus explains away the pain of suffering, but neither views sickness as a punishment from God.

Leprosy and the Purity Code

Next, let's turn to leprosy, one of those diseases that many interpreted as God's punishment. The Book of Leviticus devotes two chapters (13 and 14) to discussing this condition. The harsh rules describe an image familiar to the imaginations of many of us:

> The one who bears the sore of leprosy shall keep his garments rent and his head bare, and shall muffle his beard; he shall cry out, "Unclean, unclean!" As long as the sore is on him he shall declare himself unclean, since he is in fact unclean. He shall dwell apart, making his abode outside the camp. (13:45–46)

It is helpful to note that the biblical term often translated as "leprosy" included many forms of skin disease, including psoriasis and ringworm.

Scholars tell us that what we call leprosy today, Hansen's disease, may have entered Palestine around 300 BCE and that many of those described as lepers undoubtedly had distasteful skin diseases but not Hansen's disease.

Whatever the actual disease, these people experienced alienation and rejection. Certainly, ancient peoples were afraid of contagion, but for the people of Israel leprosy became a ritual impurity more than a medical problem. They considered it divine punishment and feared that the community would also suffer if the leper were not forced "outside the camp."

Jesus not only rejects the judgment (John 9:3) but also crosses the boundaries of purity laws to touch the alienated. Mark's Gospel describes the scene this way:

> A leper came to him [and kneeling down] begged him and said, "If you wish, you can make me clean." Moved with pity, he stretched out his hand, touched him, and said to him, "I do will it. Be made clean." The leprosy left him immediately, and he was made clean. (1:40–42)

With a simple but profound touch, Jesus breaks down barriers, challenges customs and laws that alienate, and embodies his convictions about the inclusive meaning of the reign of God. This dramatic touch is also described in the other two Synoptic Gospels, Matthew 8:1–4 and Luke 5:12–16.

This event reveals not only Jesus's care for an individual in need but also his concern about structures of society. Jesus steps across the boundaries separating the unclean and actually touches the leper. In doing so, Jesus enters into the leper's isolation and becomes unclean. Human care and compassion, not cultural values of honor and shame, direct Jesus's action. He calls into question the purity code that alienates and oppresses people already in need. Indeed, this encounter with the leper is one example of how Jesus reaches out to the marginal people in Jewish society, whether they are women, the possessed, or lepers.

Faith That Does Justice

The second biblical conviction that provides the context for developing a response to HIV/AIDS is the recognition that faith must be connected with politics, economics, and all structures of society. Even though the ancient Hebrews had a profound sense of communal life (unlike contemporary

American individualism), they too had difficulty in integrating faith into their daily lives. Again and again, the prophets challenged the people not to separate justice concerns from true religion. Isaiah powerfully expresses this conviction:

> Is this the manner of fasting I wish, of keeping a day of penance: that a man bow his head like a reed, and lie in sackcloth and ashes? Do you call this a fast, a day acceptable to the Lord? This, rather, is the fasting that I wish: releasing those bound unjustly, untying the thongs of the yoke; sharing your bread with the hungry, sheltering the oppressed and the homeless; clothing the naked when you see them, and not turning your back on your own. (Isaiah 58:5–7)

Jesus embodied and expressed this vision in his parables about God's reign and in his healings and table fellowship. His encounter with the leper is just one example; for several other examples, see Matthew 25:31–46—the final judgment, Luke 10:29–37—the Good Samaritan, and Luke 16:19–31—the rich man and the poor man.

How to Respond

Today many people suffering from HIV and AIDS experience judgment, stigmatization, and rejection—just like the leper. In ways subtle and not so subtle, they too are forced "outside the camp," whether it be housing, employment, insurance, school, or even religion. Other societal powers make the situation worse. Throughout the world, economic systems and decisions trap people in poverty. Racism fosters oppression. Religions promote judgmental attitudes. Violence and widespread denial of any real freedom force women into tragic situations. All these situations provide the perfect conditions for the spread of HIV.

How are we to respond? Clearly, our Scriptures challenge us to live as faithful disciples of Jesus. Our biblical reflections have led us to three specific points that guide responses to HIV/AIDS (as will be developed in the following chapters). (1) We resist the temptation to judge and condemn people. HIV/AIDS is not a punishment sent by God. This change of attitude is where we start. (2) We respond with care and compassion to those infected and affected by HIV, crossing the boundaries of fear and prejudice. With the attitude of Jesus, we reach out to these sisters and brothers. (3) We recognize the need for societal change as well as behavioral change. This too means action—systemic action.

Such a response accepts personal responsibility to challenge and change political platforms, economic strategies, and governmental decisions that foster a culture of oppression and death.

THE CONSISTENT ETHIC OF LIFE

A moral vision that holds together many different issues and so offers direction for action concerning the AIDS crisis is the Consistent Ethic of Life. The late Cardinal Joseph Bernardin articulated this perspective in the early 1980s, and it has become a centerpiece of the moral teaching of the Catholic bishops of the United States. Pope John Paul II affirmed similar themes in his 1995 encyclical *The Gospel of Life*. This third section uses these sources to answer three basic questions: (1) What is the Consistent Ethic of Life? (2) Where does it come from? (3) What does it mean for our everyday lives?

A Moral Framework

What is the Consistent Ethic of Life? It is a comprehensive ethical system that links together many different issues by focusing attention on the basic value of life. In his attempts to defend life, Cardinal Bernardin first joined the topics of abortion and nuclear war. He quickly expanded his understanding of a Consistent Ethic of Life to include many issues from all of life. Already in the first of a whole series of talks, Cardinal Bernardin stated: "The spectrum of life cuts across the issues of genetics, abortion, capital punishment, modern warfare and the care of the terminally ill."[13]

Cardinal Bernardin also acknowledged that issues are distinct and different; capital punishment, for example, is not the same as abortion. Nevertheless, the issues are linked. The valuing and defense of life is at the center of both issues. Cardinal Bernardin wrote: "When human life is considered 'cheap' or easily expendable in one area, eventually nothing is held as sacred and all lives are in jeopardy."[14]

Along with his consistent linking of distinct life issues, Cardinal Bernardin acknowledged that no individual or group can pursue all issues. Still, while concentrating on one issue, the individual or group must not be seen "as insensitive to or even opposed to other moral claims on the overall spectrum of life."[15] The Consistent Ethic of Life rules out contradictory moral positions about the unique value of human life—and it would be contradictory, for example, to be against abortion but for capital punishment or to work against poverty but support euthanasia. This linkage of all life issues is, of course, the very heart of the Consistent Ethic of Life. This linkage challenges us to move beyond the contradictions we may find in our own convictions about morality. Often these convictions seem to cluster around "conservative" or "liberal" viewpoints—as in the above examples. But the Consistent Ethic of Life cuts across such divisions, calling us to respect the life in the womb, the life of a criminal, the life on welfare, and the life of the dying. This moral vision, then, offers a challenging and comprehensive framework for responding to the ethical dilemmas of HIV/AIDS.

Sources of Life

Where does the Consistent Ethic of Life come from? Recent sources include the addresses and articles of Cardinal Bernardin, the teachings of the Catholic bishops of the United States, and John Paul II's encyclical *The Gospel of Life*. The ultimate source, however, is the Bible, especially the life and teaching of Jesus.

Cardinal Bernardin, because of his extensive experience in the work of the National Conference of Catholic Bishops (now called the United States Conference of Catholic Bishops), spent much time and energy on two issues: abortion and nuclear war. He found committed people concerned about one issue but not the other. As he worked to bring together those seeking an end to abortion and those trying to prevent nuclear war, Cardinal Bernardin began to emphasize the linkage among the life issues. This emphasis has been continued in the teachings of the U.S. Conference of Catholic Bishops.

Pope John Paul II's encyclical *The Gospel of Life* is another bold and prophetic defense of life. Although it does not use the phrase, *The Gospel of Life* strongly affirms the Consistent Ethic of Life. John Paul described what is going on in our world: a monumental abuse of life through drugs, war and arms, abortion, euthanasia, destruction of the environment, and unjust distribution of resources. This abuse is often caused and supported by the economic, social, and political structures of the nations. So the pope spoke of a "structure of sin" and a "culture of death" and a "conspiracy against life."[16]

The late pope also proclaimed the Christian understanding of the value of life. Created in God's image, redeemed by Jesus, called to everlasting life, every human being is sacred and social; every human being is a sign of God's love. In much more detail than Cardinal Bernardin's addresses, the pope provided the foundation for building a culture of life by weaving together a wealth of biblical texts that clearly proclaim human dignity.

The Consistent Ethic of Life is ultimately rooted in Jesus, in whom the meaning and value of life are definitively proclaimed and fully given. John Paul II stated this insight with these words: "The *Gospel of life* is not simply a reflection, however new and profound, on human life. Nor is it merely a commandment aimed at raising awareness and bringing about significant changes in society. Still less is it an illusory promise of a better future. The *Gospel of life* is something concrete and personal, for it consists in the proclamation of *the very person of Jesus*."[17]

Who is this Jesus? We have to be careful not to create Jesus in our own image. As Scripture scholar John Meier reminds us, Jesus was a "nonconformist" who associated with the religious and social outcasts. As a result of his life and teachings, Jesus "escapes all our neat categories" and is neither right nor left.[18] This is the Jesus of the Sermon on the Mount who proclaims as blessed not the leaders of society but the mourning and the meek, the poor and the pure, the persecuted and the peacemaker (Matthew 5:1–12). This is the Jesus who praises not power but reconciliation in the story about the forgiving father of the prodigal son (Luke 15:11–32). This is the Jesus of faithful ministry, of suffering and death, of new life (Mark 14:3–16:8). This is the Jesus who says, "I came that they may have life, and have it abundantly" (John 10:10). Who Jesus is and what Jesus means by abundant life, then, are surely different from what the consumerism and individualism of our culture tell us about life.

Abundant Life

What does the Consistent Ethic of Life mean for our everyday lives? (1) It encourages us to hold together a great variety of issues with a consistent focus on the value of life. (2) It challenges us to reflect on our basic values and convictions that give direction to our lives. (3) It leads us to express our commitment to life in civil debate and public policy. The combination of these three points results in an appropriate ethic for responding to HIV and AIDS.

A consistent ethic includes all life issues from the very beginning of life to its end. An excellent example of how the life ethic holds together many distinct issues is the U.S. bishops' statement on political responsibility, issued prior to every presidential election. These statements have provided direction concerning many issues, including abortion, racism, the economy, AIDS, housing, the global trade in arms, welfare reform, immigration, and refugees.

Several examples can give the spirit of this Consistent Ethic of Life. The bishops oppose the use of the death penalty, judging that the practice further undermines respect for life in our society and stating that it has been discriminatory against the poor and racial minorities. The bishops express special concern for the problem of racism, calling it a radical evil which divides the human family. Dealing with poverty, the bishops claim, is a moral imperative of the highest priority for poverty threatens life. In the domestic scene, there is a need for more jobs with adequate pay and decent working conditions; at the international level, the areas of trade, aid, and investment must be reevaluated in terms of their impact on the poor.

Capital punishment, racism, poverty: certainly these are very different issues, with different causes and different solutions (many of which may be very complex). Still, underneath all these differences is life and, for us, the challenge of respecting the lives of people who may be very different from us.

The Consistent Ethic of Life also leads us beyond the specific issues to the depths of our convictions about the meaning of life. A careful and prayerful study of the statements on political responsibility (and the more detailed teachings which they summarize) allows us to appreciate not only the expanse of the seamless garment of the Consistent Ethic of Life but also its profound challenge to our most important attitudes and values.

Emphasizing the Consistent Ethic of Life and recognizing its counter-cultural directions, the bishops state: "A Catholic moral framework does not easily fit the ideologies of 'right' or 'left,' nor the platforms of any party. Our values are often not 'politically correct.' Believers are called to be a community of conscience within the larger society and to test public life by the values of Scripture and the principles of Catholic social teaching."[19] It is not sufficient to be pro-life on some issues; we must be pro-life on all issues—no matter what our political party or business or union or talk shows or advertising or family may say. These are powerful forces that significantly shape our convictions. They often lead to the contradictions that separate us from a Consistent Ethic of Life. Politics, media, money, and class—and not our faith— may well be the real source of our values.

We ought not underestimate the challenge of being pro-life; it is so easy to justify our contradictions by appealing to common sense or accepted business practice or the ethical relativism that is our culture's morality. In *The Gospel of Life* John Paul II urged all persons to choose life—consistently, personally, nationally, and globally. This invitation is really a profound challenge: to look deeply into ourselves and to test against the Gospel some of our own deeply held beliefs and practices. John Paul writes: "In a word, we can say that the cultural change which we are calling for demands from everyone the courage to *adopt a new life-style*, consisting in making practical choices—at the personal, family, social and international level—on the basis of a correct scale of values: *the primacy of being over having, of the person over things.* This renewed lifestyle involves a passing from *indifference to concern for others, from rejection to acceptance of them.*"[20]

Cardinal Bernardin, the conference of bishops, and Pope John Paul have necessarily discussed the relationship between moral vision and political policies. Indeed, the Consistent Ethic of Life was developed to help shape public policy. Political policies and economic structures provide means to create a societal environment that promotes the flourishing of human life. "If one contends, as we do, that the right of every fetus to be born should be protected by civil law and supported by civil consensus, then our moral, political and economic responsibilities do not stop at the moment of birth. Those who defend the right to life of the weakest among us must be equally visible in support of the quality of life of the powerless among us: the old and the young, the hungry and the homeless, the undocumented immigrant and the unemployed worker. Such a quality of life posture translates into specific political and economic positions on tax policy, employment generation, welfare policy, nutrition and feeding programs, and health care."[21]

During the past one hundred years, bishops and popes have addressed issues of politics and economics in their social teachings. Key themes from this tradition include human dignity, solidarity, justice, and the common good.

Human dignity is the foundation of all the social teachings. This theme is discussed in detail in two documents: Blessed Pope John XXIII's *Peace on Earth* and Vatican II's *The Church in the Modern World*. Because all human beings are created in God's image, we are sacred and precious. Accordingly, all persons have worth and dignity, rooted simply in who they are (and not in what they do or achieve). Situations that limit or undermine human dignity cry out for change. All forms of discrimination are wrong, whether in housing, jobs, insurance, health care, or religion.

Technology and globalization constantly remind us of the deeper interdependence of the human family. Many of Pope John Paul II's writings emphasized this solidarity, especially with the poor of the world. He affirmed that the Church follows God in expressing a preferential option for the poor. This option recognizes the power of economic and social structures to perpetuate poverty and limit personal freedom, harming both those who oppress and those who are oppressed. The pope named such conditions "structures of sin" in his 1987 encyclical *On Social Concern*.[22]

Justice, right relationships along with the structural recognition of human dignity and rights and responsibilities, is another major theme emphasized throughout the social teachings. The Synod of Bishops in 1971 described the massive divisions in the world between rich and poor and called for justice for all. In a celebrated passage in the Synod's *Justice in the World*, the bishops declare: "Action on behalf of justice and participation in the transformation of the world appear to us as a constitutive dimension of the preaching of the gospel."[23]

The goal of justice is to create a global society where the common good flourishes. The common good, according to John XXIII in *Peace on Earth*, means all those things necessary for all peoples to live truly human lives. What most of us take for granted—food, water, clothing, shelter, sanitation, appropriate health care, and participation in politics—is lacking in the lives of hundreds of millions of the human family.

As Cardinal Bernardin realized, we must also be able to state our case "in non-religious terms which others of different faith convictions might find morally persuasive."[24] For example, we may be opposed to euthanasia and assisted suicide fundamentally because of our faith convictions about God as giver of the gift of life and about our own stewardship of life. For public policy discussion, however, we may stress other reasons, such as human dignity, the undermining of trust in the medical profession, and the threat to women and the vulnerable.

Church teachings emphasize that faithfulness to the Gospel leads not only to individual acts of charity but also to actions involving the institutions and structures of society, the economy, and politics. The bishops of the United States, for example, state: "We encourage people to use their voices and votes to enrich the democratic life of our nation and to act on their values in the political arena. We hope American Catholics, as both believers *and* citizens, will use the resources of our faith and the opportunities of this democracy to help shape a society more respectful of the life, dignity, and rights of the human person, especially the poor and vulnerable."[25] Clearly, religion and politics must mix in our lives! We face the challenge of embodying consistently an ethic of life in the candidates we support and in our own direct involvement in forming public policy.

ETHICS AND AIDS

As we enter a new millennium, world events and Church teachings direct our attention to life itself as the very center of our concern. The Consistent Ethic of Life provides both a solid foundation and a powerful challenge to live as faithful disciples and involved citizens. It calls into question all views that contradict the message and meaning of Jesus. It challenges us to reject the culture of death and to create a culture of life in and through our everyday activities at home and at work and in society.

The Consistent Ethic of Life urges us to speak and act not only concerning abortion and euthanasia but also concerning welfare and immigration, sexism and racism, maximization of profits and health-care reform, trade agreements and sweatshops, the buying and selling of women for prostitution, genocide, and many other issues—all connected to HIV and AIDS (as will be discussed in the following chapters). Based on ancient Scriptures and attentive to contemporary experiences, the Consistent Ethic of Life provides an ethical framework for confronting the moral dilemmas raised by HIV and AIDS and for promoting the full flourishing of all life. And so we turn to the five clusters of moral issues that were briefly described in the Introduction.

NOTES

1. Richard M. Gula, S.S., *Reason Informed by Faith: Foundations of Catholic Morality* (Mahwah, N.J.: Paulist Press, 1989), 1–5.

2. James M. Gustafson, *Protestant and Roman Catholic Ethics: Prospects for Rapprochement* (Chicago: The University of Chicago Press, 1978), 30–59.

3. John F. Kavanaugh, S.J., *(Still) Following Christ in a Consumer Society* (Maryknoll, N.Y.: Orbis Books, 1991), 105–15.

4. John W. Crossin, *What Are They Saying about Virtue?* (Mahwah, N.J.: Paulist Press, 1985), 13–52.

5. John P. Galvin, "The Invitation of Grace" in *A World of Grace,* ed. Leo J. O'Donovan (New York: The Crossroad Publishing Company, 1987), 64–91.

6. Marcus J. Borg, *Meeting Jesus Again for the First Time* (New York: HarperCollins Publishers, 1994), 68, note 50.

7. Pope John Paul II, *The Gospel of Life* (Boston: Pauline Books & Media, 1995), 19–44.

8. Michael D. Guinan, O.F.M., *To Be Human before God* (Collegeville, Minn.: The Liturgical Press, 1994), 46–60.

9. Karl Rahner, S.J., "The Dignity and Freedom of Man," *Theological Investigations*, Vol. II (Baltimore: Helicon Press, 1963), 235–64.

10. Gula, *Reason*, 265–82.

11. Timothy E. O'Connell, *Principles for a Catholic Morality,* rev. ed. (New York: HarperCollins Publishers, 1990), 109–14.

12. O'Connell, *Catholic Morality*, 186.

13. Joseph Cardinal Bernardin, *Consistent Ethic of Life* (Kansas City: Sheed & Ward, 1988), 7.

14. Bernardin, *Consistent Ethic*, 89.

15. Bernardin, *Consistent Ethic*, 15.

16. John Paul II, *Gospel of Life*, para.12, 27.

17. John Paul II, *Gospel of Life,* para. 29, 52.

18. John Meier, "Jesus," in *The New Jerome Biblical Commentary,* eds. Raymond Brown, S.S., Joseph Fitzmeyer, S.J., and Roland Murphy, O.Carm (Englewood Cliffs, N.J.: Prentice Hall, 1990), 1316–28, at 1318.

19. Administrative Committee of the U.S. Conference of Catholic Bishops, "Faithful Citizenship," *Origins* 33, no. 20 (23 October 2003): 324.

20. John Paul II, *Gospel of Life*, para. 98, 154.

21. Bernardin, *Consistent Ethic*, 8–9.

22. Pope John Paul II, *On Social Concern* (Washington, D.C.: USCC Office of Publishing Services, 1987), para. 36, 69.

23. Second Synod of Bishops, "Justice in the World," in *The Gospel of Peace and Justice*, ed. Joseph Gremillion (Maryknoll, N.Y.: Orbis Books, 1976), 514.

24. Bernardin, *Consistent Ethic*, 10.

25. USCC Administrative Board, "Political Responsibility," *Origins* 25, no. 22 (16 November 1995): 374.

Chapter Three

Ethics and the Beginning of Life

HIV and AIDS raise ethical questions that extend throughout the life cycle and around the globe. In this chapter, we will consider some of those linked to the beginning of life: birth, infancy, and childhood. (1) Ought HIV-infected women avoid becoming pregnant? (2) What methods to prevent HIV transmission ought to be used? (3) Could abortion ever be justified? (4) What is the proper treatment for HIV-infected infants and children? (5) What is society's responsibility for care of AIDS orphans?

The Consistent Ethic of Life provides the moral framework for searching for answers to these questions. An essential element of this search must always be the focus on structural influences that limit personal choices.

HIV-INFECTED WOMEN AND PREGNANCY

Ought HIV-infected women avoid becoming pregnant? Of course, as we know from UN statistics, a significant percentage of HIV-positive people do not know that they are infected. Also, in many situations, the oppression of women (see chapter 7) often reduces or eliminates the possibility of choice. This first question, then, is limited, but still significant.

What facts are involved in this situation? For an HIV-positive woman who does not receive any kind of treatment and who breastfeeds her child, there is about a 30 percent chance that the child will become infected.

With timely and appropriate treatment with preventive drugs, this percentage can be reduced to as low as 2 percent. In many areas where the epidemic is very bad, only 5 percent of HIV-infected pregnant women have access to any treatment, although the number of women receiving services has risen over the past couple of years.[1] Maximum reduction of mother to child transmission depends on identifying HIV infection as early as possible during pregnancy and the woman and her newborn receiving the proper preventive drugs and AIDS treatment.

Strategies for the prevention of mother to child transmission that have been shown to be effective have increased dramatically since the late 1990s. The primary strategy (in addition to avoidance of breastfeeding) is the use of the antiretroviral zidovudine (ZDV) administered to the mother during the second and third trimesters of pregnancy, labor and delivery, and to the newborn after birth. Other effective strategies to reduce the risk of transmission involve short-course regimens using ZDV and other antiretrovirals, beginning as late as the onset of labor and possibly antiretroviral treatment only of the newborn. The risk of transmission is reduced among breastfeeding and nonbreastfeeding women alike, although efficacy is lower in the latter. Among breastfeeding African women, the antiretroviral nevirapine (NVP) has been shown to be highly effective and very popular due to lower cost and ease of administration. It is given as a single dose to the HIV-infected woman in labor and to the infant within seventy-two hours of birth.

Reducing exposure of the infant to infected maternal blood and secretions during labor and delivery by elective cesarean section can also prevent HIV transmission. However, in resource-poor countries, this procedure, if available at all, may present its own risks for the mother and newborn. Interventions promoted in many countries of the developing world also include the use of less invasive medical procedures during childbirth, safe infant feeding practices as alternatives to breastfeeding, and prevention and treatment of malaria.

Researchers have shown that high viral load in the pregnant woman increases the likelihood of transmission of the virus to the newborn. They emphasize, as a result, the importance of the provision of effective antiretroviral treatment for the health of the mother in order to reduce mother to child transmission. Although pregnancy itself will affect the timing and choice of antiretroviral treatment, and many unanswered questions remain about these and other issues, researchers generally agree that the benefits of antiretroviral treatment outweigh the risks.[2]

Medical issues often raise moral questions. For example, as indicated above, the short course treatment of nevirapine is especially popular in resource-poor countries. Now, however, recent studies have indicated that the mother may have fewer treatment options in the future because resistance to nevirapine or related drugs can easily develop in this treatment. At the time of the writing of this chapter, both the medical and the moral debates continued concerning the problematic use of nevirapine.

Children have long been seen as a blessing of marriage, even the purpose of it. So the Consistent Ethic of Life would clearly support this affirmation of life. Still questions must be asked. In resource-poor situations, the possibility of giving birth to an infected child is much higher. Moreover, the likelihood that the mother will die in the near future (because of the lack of treatment resources) intensifies the negative dimensions of the situation. What future awaits the child, even if the child survives without being infected? While it certainly does not seem appropriate to see avoidance of pregnancy as the only moral choice, it must at least be recognized as a possible option.

As noted earlier, we must also look to the political and economic realities, especially poverty and oppression, that put women in this dilemma. Many moral issues emerge, such as the lack of counseling and testing, stigmatization, inadequate alternatives to breastfeeding, and lack of medical care, especially antiretroviral treatment for the mother. Here the moral choice is clear: to change the structures that limit treatment possibilities (more on this in chapter 7). This first question about pregnancy leads naturally to the second.

METHODS TO PREVENT HIV TRANSMISSION

What methods to prevent HIV transmission ought to be used? Specifically, in the context of this discussion, can condoms be used? How are condoms to be described: as contraception or a means to protect life? This combination of questions has generated more reactions than probably any other question, especially in the Roman Catholic Church.

Some of the roots of this present debate can be found in the earlier discussion surrounding Pope Paul VI's 1968 encyclical, *Humanae Vitae*, in which the pope wrote that all forms of artificial contraception were morally wrong.[3] Many theologians (and others) argued that a more person-centered[4] interpretation of natural law would yield a different judgment. This "order of reason" approach emphasized the whole person-in-relation rather than biological aspects of a specific act in determining the morality of the act.[5]

Not surprisingly then, a new round of discussions developed after the Administrative Board of the United States Catholic Conference issued *The Many Faces of AIDS* in 1987. In this pastoral statement, the bishops summarized church teaching about sexuality and then cautiously acknowledged that not all people would follow this teaching and so should receive information about condoms.[6] After the publication of the document, others objected to this reference to condoms. Another statement, *Called to Compassion and Responsibility*, was issued two years later from the whole conference of bishops, in which official Church teaching on human sexuality was emphasized.[7]

Because of the increasing evidence that the use of condoms can be an effective means of preventing the spread of HIV/AIDS and because of the growing split between the official teaching and many people working in AIDS clinics,[8] new theological reflections have again engaged the question. James Keenan, S.J., has edited *Catholic Ethicists on HIV/AIDS Prevention* that attempts to draw on various resources in the Catholic tradition to address effective HIV prevention.

In the spirit of *The Many Faces of AIDS*, Cardinal Godfried Danneels of Mechelen-Brussels in a 2004 interview reaffirmed Catholic teaching about sexual activity only in marriage and abstinence as a protection against HIV infection. Then he added that if an infected person disregards abstinence, then that person ought to protect the other by using a condom, so that the individual not also violate the Fifth Commandment, "You shall not kill."[9]

Similarly, some French and African bishops have claimed that, in a situation where one spouse is HIV-positive, use of a condom could be considered as a means to avoid a life-threatening disease, not as a contraceptive.[10]

The Consistent Ethic of Life certainly supports the efforts to extend effective HIV prevention. The fundamental cause of the condom debate, however, is to be found primarily in the interpretation of natural law. While the more holistic emphasis of the Consistent Ethic would seem to fit better with the modern worldview and its order of reason,[11] the differences of interpretation are not likely to be resolved easily. Each of the two sides has become quite convinced of the correctness of its position. The tension will remain.[12]

ABORTION

Could abortion ever be justified? Here is another emotional, much debated topic. As in other difficult situations, the choice for abortion in the context of AIDS is understandable. Fear for the status and future of the child and/or concern for the mother's own health and future could lead to the decision to abort.

As noted above, however, the possibility of giving birth to a noninfected child is greater than the possibility of an HIV-positive child. With treatment, the possibility is even greater. Still, in the majority of situations medical treatment is not available for the mother, so her chances of seeing her child become a teenager are very low.

That abortion is an understandable choice, of course, does not necessarily make it a moral choice. Indeed, the Consistent Ethic of Life was first developed in the context of the abortion debate and the Catholic Church's strong opposition to abortion.[13] Official Church teaching considers every abortion to be morally wrong.[14]

Many who support the consistent life ethic also find a few situations in which abortion might be justified (in light of the discerning methodology described in chapter 2).[15] For example, in an ectopic pregnancy the new life begins to develop in the fallopian tube, with no chance of survival. The situation is also a threat to the mother. An older moral methodology using the principle of the double-effect[16] would justify the removal of the fallopian tube with the new life in it. But with modern science, the fallopian tube can now be shelled out (by technology or drug), thus saving the mother but performing (technically) an abortion. Given the real balance of act, intention, circumstances, and consequences,[17] the discerning methodology would justify the decision to preserve life by taking life.[18]

Similar arguments might be made in other situations where the mother's life is at risk.[19] It is not clear, however, that HIV/AIDS results in such a direct risk. As we saw in the first question of this chapter, an infected mother can still continue to receive her drug therapy (HAART) if it is available. Clearly, in many situations in the world, the child will face both the death of the mother and an uncertain future. Here, the Consistent Ethic of Life affirms that even this uncertainty is to be chosen rather than certain death. Again, this very personal decision points to societal issues of health care, poverty, and care for orphans (and it can be noted that maternal mortality is already very high in many places, even without HIV/AIDS—pointing to the urgency of facing these systemic issues). Rather than turn to violence, society must search for creative, life-affirming ways to confront difficulties and conflicts.[20]

TREATMENT FOR HIV-INFECTED
INFANTS AND CHILDREN

What is the proper treatment for HIV-infected infants and children? As we saw in the first question of this chapter, even minimal prophylactic treatment reduces the risk of an HIV-positive mother giving birth to an infected child. Still, the World Health Organization estimates that there were seven hundred thousand children under the age of fifteen newly infected in 2005, most in the birthing process. UNAIDS/WHO also estimates that five hundred seventy thousand children died from AIDS in 2005, most in resource-limited countries.[21]

A 2004 survey reveals startling numbers for South Africa. According to this study, almost 7 percent of children between the ages of two and nine are HIV-positive, much higher than expected.[22]

Lack of treatment, of course, is the real issue. With the movement to provide antiretroviral drugs slowly growing, some countries are now making this therapy available for some children. The result is dramatic, with the children not only surviving but thriving.[23] Long-term questions remain concerning both the efficacy of the drugs (possible issues of resistance, etc.) and the availability of the therapy when they are no longer children.

The more general topic of treatment of infants received extensive medical and ethical attention in the 1980s. The case that caused this attention took place in Bloomington, Indiana. Parents of a newborn baby with Down's syndrome and a condition that prevented the ingestion of food barred doctors from treating the baby, who, of course, then died.

In response, the U.S. government issued several statements outlawing discrimination against handicapped infants.

Ethicists, while opposed to the parents' decision, tried to develop more nuanced guidelines (because in some situations nontreatment might be a moral choice).[24] Richard McCormick, S.J., proposed the following: "(1) Lifesaving interventions ought not to be omitted for institutional or managerial reasons. . . . However, it remains an unacceptable erosion of our respect for life to make the gift of life once given depend on the emotions or financial capacities of the parents alone."[25] Then, significantly, especially for our present consideration of HIV/AIDS, he concludes: "At this point society has some responsibilities."[26] McCormick adds an editorial footnote: "It is sad and even inconsistent that the very administration that insists that handicapped infants be treated is the one drastically reducing the funds to make this care possible."[27]

McCormick's other three points are: "(2) Lifesaving interventions may not be omitted simply because the baby is retarded," but (3) "may be omitted or withdrawn when there is excessive hardship, especially when this combines with poor prognosis" or (4) "when it becomes clear that expected life can be had only for a relatively brief time and only with the continued use of artificial feeding."[28]

McCormick's guidelines summarize well the Catholic tradition's directions for end-of-life treatments. Ethically ordinary means must be used; ethically extraordinary means are optional. Ethically ordinary means are medicines or treatments that offer a reasonable hope of benefit and can be used without excessive pain, expense, or other inconvenience. Ethically extraordinary means do not offer reasonable hope of benefit or include excessive pain, expense, or other inconvenience (see also chapter 5).[29]

For HIV-infected infants, so much depends on the situation into which they are born. This issue is usually the availability of treatment rather than parental choice. Where choice is a true option, the guidelines offer sound direction. Evidence clearly indicates the benefit of drug therapy, though there is the issue of cost. Especially concerning this point, McCormick's note about society's responsibilities deserves close attention. Perhaps, then, the more pressing moral question becomes: How much effort must be put into effective treatment of HIV-infected infants and children?

In the real world at this time, however, the great percentage of HIV-infected infants will only receive minimal comfort care as their disease progresses.

ORPHANS

What is society's responsibility for care of AIDS orphans? The AIDS epidemic has already created millions of orphans. UNAIDS/WHO defines an orphan as a child who, before the age of fifteen, lost either one's mother or both parents. The survey mentioned in the last question adds some specifics for South Africa: Almost 10 percent of the children aged two to nine had a parent die; for the fifteen to eighteen age group, it was 25 percent. Three percent of children aged twelve to eighteen considered themselves head of the family.[30]

In the developing world, children are particularly vulnerable to the impact of the epidemic. Indeed, most aspects of their lives—food, education, sexuality, family life, life itself—are threatened. Even before they become orphans, when children have parents with AIDS, they face growing problems that are often overlooked in the epidemic. Because the family's scarce resources are spread even more thinly for various needs, the children often receive less food, may have to leave school to work, and face stigma and marginalization. Many cultures still resist discussion and education about sexuality, resulting in greater risk for the children. With the death of the parent(s), these and other threats intensify, including dealing with the psychological trauma of their parent's death.

Although in many cultures the extended family traditionally takes in the orphans, this tradition is weakening, perhaps because of fear and prejudice or simply because of the lack of resources in the context of so many orphans. Because so many young adults are dying, grandparents face the impossible task of raising and caring for perhaps dozens of their grandchildren.

Most countries with extensive epidemics still do not have sufficient programs to provide appropriate care for orphans.[31] As a result, many of the orphans cannot be cared for by extended families and so end up on the street. They face "psychological suffering, deprivation, social exclusion, and multiple health risks."[32] Many leave school in order to work. Girls are more likely to become sexually active at a younger age. Orphans confront the stigma and discrimination connected to HIV/AIDS: studies have shown that other orphans fare better than AIDS orphans.[33]

The massive work, *AIDS in the World*, summarizes all these threats to the flourishing of life this way: "Sadly, those children most vulnerable to HIV infection—victims of sexual abuse, street children, those sold into sex work, the children of sex workers, and young girls whose cultures and societies deny them the right to say no to males—are also most likely to be deprived of the information, education, and support that could help them avoid infection with HIV."[34]

Clearly, resources are the key issue once again. If antiretroviral drug therapy were available for the parents, then the children would not become orphans. A whole chain of results could be avoided, saving costs in so many ways. Treatment, then, along with continuing efforts at prevention, becomes the key response.

Nevertheless, the reality of millions of orphans deserves immediate response, beginning with basic education for everyone. Clearly, such a response will be extremely difficult to fashion. The difficulties abound; here are two foundational ones. In most countries, some cultural patterns increase the risk of infection for children, for example, the lack of childhood education about sex and sexuality and gender-based inequities. Although there is no easy way to change such social traditions, political and religious leadership can make a difference, especially when the necessary information is presented in culturally and religiously sensitive ways.[35]

In resource-wealthy countries, a very different kind of cultural tradition is equally challenging: commitment to particular economic worldviews and structures (more on this in chapters 6 and 7). Promoting solidarity and the common good would transform these worldviews and structures, with implications not only for the care of orphans but for the entire response to the HIV/AIDS epidemic.

Concerning this just allocation of resources and orphans, Stephen Lewis, UN special envoy for HIV/AIDS in Africa, boldly states: "We know what it means to find a way of integrating orphans back into the community when their parents have died. We have all over the continent individual projects and programmes that are successful."[36] What is needed is political will, leadership, reorientation of values, and redistribution of resources.

These five questions concerning the beginning of life have revealed that the Consistent Ethic of Life, embodying the social teaching's themes of dignity, solidarity, justice, and the common good, offers a comprehensive moral framework for addressing complex ethical dilemmas. Human life is a basic but not absolute good. By one's very existence, a human being deserves respect and an ever-widening circle of rights and responsibilities. The authentic flourishing of life begins with life itself and spills over into food, family life, education, and so many other aspects of life lived in community. Almost every one of these aspects is threatened by HIV/AIDS, from life in the womb to life impacted by economic structures. The defense and promotion of life, then, demands individual, communal, and global transformation— from a culture of death to a culture of life!

NOTES

1. UNAIDS and the World Health Organization, "AIDS Epidemic Update," *UNAIDS*, www.unaids.org/Epi2005/doc/EPIupdate2005_pdf_en/epi-update2005_en.pdf 13 (accessed 19 December 2005).

2. Julian Meldrum, "Preventing Mother to Child Transmission of HIV," *NAM*, www.aidsmap.com/en/docs/1A3EDD95-C60B-4BFF-83D 5-CE706AA88191.asp (accessed 1 July 2004).

3. Richard A. McCormick, S.J., *Notes on Moral Theology 1965 through 1980* (Washington, D.C.: University Press of America, 1981), 38–52, 109–16, 164–68, 208–31, 233–43, 768–85.

4. Richard M. Gula, S.S., *Reason Informed by Faith: Foundations of Catholic Morality* (Mahwah, N.J.: Paulist Press, 1989), 242–46.

5. Gula, *Reason*, 32–33, 242–46.

6. Administrative Board of the United States Catholic Conference, *The Many Faces of AIDS: A Gospel Response* (Washington, D.C.: USCC Office of Publishing Services, 1987), 18.

7. Jon D. Fuller, S.J., and James F. Keenan, S.J., "Introduction: At the End of the First Generation of HIV Prevention," in *Catholic Ethicists on HIV/AIDS Prevention*, ed. James F. Keenan, S.J. (New York: Continuum, 2002), 21–25.

8. Fuller and Keenan, "Introduction," 21–25; see also UNAIDS, "Epidemic Update," 12.

9. Editors, "Signs of the Times," *America* 190, no. 3 (2 February 2004): 5.

10. Editors, "Signs," 5; see also Laurie Goering, "A Two-front Fight: AIDS, the Church," *Chicago Tribune*, 4 November 2005, 1, 16; for contexts other than discordant couples, it must be noted that recent evidence (UNAIDS, "Epidemic Update," 25–27) shows that HIV infection rates have been brought down by delay of the first sexual encounter and reducing the number of sexual partners (see chapter 6 for the ABC approach).

11. Gula, *Reason,* 32–33.

12. Richard A. McCormick, S.J., "The Consistent Ethic of Life: Is There an Historical Soft Underbelly?" in *Consistent Ethic of Life*, Joseph Cardinal Bernardin (Kansas City: Sheed and Ward, 1988), 97–104; Gula, *Reason*, 231–49.

13. Joseph Cardinal Bernardin, "A Consistent Ethic of Life: An American-Catholic Dialogue," in *Consistent Ethic*, 1–26.

14. The Holy See, *Catechism of the Catholic Church* (Liguori, Mo.: Liguori Publications, 1994), no. 2271.

15. McCormick, "Soft Underbelly?" 109–12.

16. Gula, *Reason*, 270–72; McCormick, *Notes 1965 through 1980*, 711–23.

17. Russell B. Connors Jr. and Patrick T. McCormick, *Character, Choices, & Community: The Three Faces of Christian Ethics* (Mahwah, N.J.: Paulist Press, 1998), 47–53.

18. Gula, S.S., *Reason*, 270–73.

19. Richard A. McCormick, S.J., *Corrective Vision: Explorations in Moral Theology* (Kansas City: Sheed and Ward, 1994), 189–200.

20. Joseph Cardinal Bernardin, *A Moral Vision for America*, edited by John P. Langan, S.J. (Washington, D.C.: Georgetown University Press, 1998), 79–92.

21. UNAIDS, "Epidemic Update," 2.

22. Keith Alcorn, "Impact of HIV on South African Children Underestimated," quoting the report of Dr. Olive Shisana of the South African Human Sciences Research Council, *NAM*, www.aidsmap.com/en/news/69A02207 -BF63-489B-87E9-11CE857DACFB.asp (accessed 6 July 2004).

23. Author's observation during visit to AIDS orphanage in Lima, Peru, in 2004.

24. Richard A. McCormick, S.J., *Notes on Moral Theology 1981 through 1984* (Lanham, Md.: University Press of America, 1984), 152–55.

25. McCormick, *Notes 1981 through 1984*, 155.

26. McCormick, *Notes 1981 through 1984*, 155.

27. McCormick, *Notes 1981 through 1984*, 119.

28. McCormick, *Notes 1981 through 1984*, 155.

29. The Congregation for the Doctrine of the Faith, *Declaration on Euthanasia* (Washington, D.C.: USCC Office of Publishing Services, 1980).

30. Alcorn, "Impact on Children," 1.

31. UNAIDS and the World Health Organization, "AIDS Epidemic Update 2003," *UNAIDS*, www.unaids.org/EN/other/functionalities/Search.asp 4 (accessed 20 December 2005).

32. Alexander Irwin, Joyce Millen, and Dorothy Fallows, *Global AIDS: Myths and Facts* (Cambridge, Mass.: South End Press, 2003), 144.

33. Irwin, Millen, and Fallows, *Global AIDS*, 145.

34. Mike Bailey, "Children and AIDS," in *AIDS in the World*, eds. Jonathan Mann, Daniel J. M. Tarantola, and Thomas W. Netter (Cambridge, Mass: Harvard University Press, 1992), 671.

35. Laurenti Magesa, "Recognizing the Reality of African Religion in Tanzania," in *Catholic Ethicists on HIV/AIDS Prevention*, ed. James F. Keenan, S.J. (New York: Continuum, 2002), 76–84.

36. Quoted in *Global AIDS*, 181–82.

Chapter Four

Ethics and Relationships

HIV and AIDS raise ethical questions that extend throughout the life cycle and around the globe. In this chapter, we will consider some of those related to HIV-infected persons and their relationships. (1) What are their moral responsibilities concerning risky behavior that could infect others? (2) Must they inform current and past sex and drug injecting partners? (3) How do HIV-discordant couples decide about their sexual behavior? (4) What about dealings with health-care providers: issues of privacy, confidentiality, truth-telling, and using experimental drugs?

These and other questions about relationships surfaced early on in the epidemic, always in variations depending on the availability of resources and on cultural values and structures. Because of the initial (and continuing) problem of stigmatization, great attention was given to issues of confidentiality, society's conflicting responsibilities, and traditional responses to epidemics. In the United States and other developed countries, affected groups were successful for the most part in protecting privacy and formulating practices that attempted to limit disclosure of one's status. The spread of the epidemic has resulted in pressures to change some of these practices.

RESPONSIBILITIES OF HIV-INFECTED PERSONS

What are the responsibilities of HIV-infected persons concerning risky behavior that could infect others? This question is again deserving of special concern because recent studies in several countries indicate that infected persons are having more unprotected sex.[1] In the late 1990s, after the use of HAART began, there was a decrease in the rate of infection in some countries. A troubling increase, however, returned in 2000. Studies indicate that HAART may reduce infectivity by 60 percent, yet incidence of infection now remains stable, the result of more unprotected sex.[2]

Researchers suggest several possible reasons for the increase in unprotected sex. First is what they call "safer sex fatigue." Persons have grown tired of taking precautions and so return to old habits and practices. Second, the success of HAART has led some to believe that HIV is less serious, that it can be treated effectively.[3]

At least one recent study offers a twist on this last reason, that because of concern for side effects or questions about long-term toleration, people are using HAART less consistently.[4] The study cautions about the possibility of a resurgent HIV epidemic.

Other researchers present a similar concern. Their study indicates that the use of methamphetamine is particularly popular with urban gay men.[5] Besides its harmful and addictive properties and its impact on the immune system, methamphetamine also impairs judgment and so leads to unprotected sex and to increased possibilities of infection. The use of meth may also lead to missing doses of HAART, possibly resulting in the development of drug resistant strains of HIV and in faster progression of the disease.[6]

These examples come from studies dealing primarily with gay men in the developed world. What about other contexts? Among young Canadian drug users, women and persons of First Nation origin are at particular risk of co-infection with HIV and hepatitis C.[7] Women throughout the world are at risk—from their infected husbands, from survival sex (trading sex for money, food, and school fees), and from a host of cultural and social factors.

In her book, *Women in the Time of AIDS*, Gillian Paterson tells the stories of several women, including Shunila from Bangladesh. Married at fifteen to a distant cousin she hardly knew, Shunila gave birth to three girls before she was twenty, when her husband (who had another wife) threw her and the girls out of the house. Perceived as a disgrace, she survived with her daughters on the streets for three months, in part by having sex for money to buy food. Eventually, she learned of a shelter for abandoned or battered women. Later she learned that she had AIDS, perhaps from her truck-driver husband or encounters on the street.[8]

Paterson asks what killed Shunila. The virus? Immorality? Paterson points to "the whole complex range of factors that govern the infrastructure of many poor women's lives."[9] Factors such as poverty, lack of education, subordination and low social status, and little freedom.[10]

Such "Third World" stories also take place in the United States, not only in urban centers but in an alarming way in the rural South. Here new cases among African-Americans account for almost two-thirds of all new cases. Dahleen Glanton writes: "In a striking parallel to the AIDS epidemic in Africa, HIV is sweeping through black communities in the South, where stigma, inadequate medical care and poverty hamper efforts to educate and prevent its spread."[11]

Glanton's article includes the story of DeShala Thompson who was infected at age seventeen by her twenty-nine-year-old boyfriend. They had planned to marry. She later found out that besides dating women, he also had sex with men. She claims that he knew he was HIV-positive but did not tell her. He infected five other women before he died.[12]

Raising our first question in this context of complexity, then, is clearly most appropriate. What are the responsibilities of HIV-infected persons concerning risky behavior that could infect others? As we saw in chapter 2, the fact of our being "body people" points to the moral obligation to care for our bodies. The Consistent Ethic of Life, of course, applies this responsibility not only to our own life but to others as well. Accordingly, HIV-infected persons ought to use appropriate means to prevent infecting others. Not doing drugs or not sharing dirty needles would fit this norm. So would sexual abstinence. We also saw in chapter 3 that some people consider condom use to be such life-preserving means (rather than contraception). As the above examples indicate, however, in situations of oppression and poverty such care for life is often not a particular value for an individual. This view is understandable and real, but not healthy or moral. "Fatigue" is not a sufficient reason for failure to care for another's life, nor is trust in new medications.

Given the pervasive influence of social structures, appeal to personal responsibility is important but not sufficient. Changing the social and cultural influences that promote irresponsibility must also receive attention, especially those that support male domination (as stressed by Paterson and many others). Culturally sensitive programs that empower women socially and economically are essential for stopping the spread of the virus.[13]

INFORMING PARTNERS

Must HIV-infected persons inform current and past sex and drug injecting partners? This question highlights a long debate about and tension between public health and privacy. According to laws in many areas, some diseases are considered "reportable diseases." Medical personnel are required by law to report certain infections, such as syphilis and gonorrhea, to a public health department. This practice is called mandatory reporting. In many places it is coupled with the follow-up process of contact tracing, more frequently referred to now as partner notification. Partner notification involves working with an infected person to identify, locate, and inform other persons ("contacts") that they may have been exposed to infection through sex or needle sharing with someone recently found to have that infection. The infected person's identity is not revealed to the other persons. These persons are then encouraged to be tested for the infection and, if found to be infected, to avoid spreading it to others.

For many years now, public health officials have found this method of detecting transmission of infectious diseases to be an important response to epidemics. It has led to treatment when necessary and to awareness and prevention—and so to protecting public health.

Mandatory reporting and partner notification puts a higher value on the common good of the public health than on individual rights to privacy. Rarely in the United States do we find the balance tipping toward the protection of the group rather than toward the protection of individual decision-making, but this is one of those situations.

Because of the reality of discrimination and stigmatization toward HIV-positive persons early in the epidemic, activists urged that HIV/AIDS not be a reportable disease. Anonymous testing allows for individuals to find out their status, with positive results being reported with no names attached. Activists (and others) argued that this anonymous testing would, in fact, encourage more people to be tested, and so would do more for limiting the spread of HIV (presuming that knowledge of one's positive status would translate into responsible behavior).

On the other hand, mandatory name-based reporting would drive people away from testing, in fear of discrimination and stigmatization, should their positive status become known.

Others, especially many in public health, argue that mandatory reporting and partner notification not only provide much more information in understanding the epidemic but also save people's lives by treatment and prevention. Especially with the newer antiretroviral treatment, this perspective has convinced more and more people and led to changes in the law in many states in the United States and elsewhere. In every state in the United States, health workers must report AIDS cases to the Centers for Disease Control and Prevention (CDC). All states also report cases of HIV infection, many with confidential name-based reporting, others with some type of code rather than the person's name.[14] The CDC now recommends that all states use the name-based reporting, noting that personal identifiers are removed before the information is given to the CDC. Still, the possibility of the breach of confidentiality, with its resulting discrimination, remains a serious concern.[15]

As we saw in the first question, the Consistent Ethic of Life affirms the individual's responsibility to prevent harm to one's self or to others by avoiding risky behavior. Concern for the other easily extends to informing those who may have been infected when, in fact, risky behavior was engaged in. This allows them the opportunity to seek out testing and treatment, if necessary, and to make decisions about future actions.

Embodying this responsibility in civil law is a more complex issue. Given the continuing presence of discrimination (to be discussed in more detail in chapter 6), the debate between public health and privacy, between epidemiologists and activists, must be taken seriously. Carefully researched studies on significant dimensions of the question could offer sound direction: does mandatory name-based reporting of HIV infection and partner notification effectively reduce the number of infections? Or do these practices drive people away from testing? In the long run, does anonymous testing actually reduce infections? Or is this practice simply the result of political pressure by groups with influence? Can motivations be determined for laws concerning partner notification: fear or punishment or good public health medicine? Is there a way to separate ideology from sound judgment?

The Consistent Ethic of Life, with its roots in the social teachings' emphasis on the common good, certainly holds on to the possibility of mandatory name-based reporting and contact tracing as a means to promote human flourishing. At the same time, its roots in the tradition's strong affirmation of the dignity of human beings leads to support of individual rights and responsibilities, and so to support of anonymous testing. Similarly, the Consistent Ethic would reject laws primarily rooted in prejudice.

As more places implement mandatory name-based reporting and especially partner notification, careful analysis of the results may clarify this dilemma and indicate which practice better promotes the flourishing of life.

DECISIONS ABOUT SEXUAL BEHAVIOR

How do HIV-discordant couples decide about their sexual behavior? Lizzie Porter was seventeen when she was diagnosed with HIV, the result of unprotected sex with a man in his thirties. She reports that she was also being abused by her stepfather at the time. Though infected, she did not get any medical care. Later she married and believes that she infected her husband. She states that he knew that she was HIV-positive but did not use any protection. She adds, "He loves me and chose to have sex without a condom. I guess I could have said 'no' more forcibly, but I decided that it was his life and choice."[16]

Globally, motivations and the availability of resources vary greatly. We have already seen that in many situations and cultures women have little freedom concerning sexual relations in marriage. We have already discussed official Catholic teaching and the use of condoms. For discordant couples (when one spouse is HIV-positive), is a condom contraceptive or life-preserving?

Ignorance, poverty, drugs, and being overwhelmed with other issues may lead to a surprising lack of interest about protection (as in Lizzie Porter's husband's case, perhaps). In such situations, how does one balance love and desire with caution and care, along with all these other factors?

In chapter 1 we heard a striking comment from Pope John Paul II. "The threat of AIDS now confronts our generations with the end of earthly life in a manner which is all the more overwhelming because it is linked, directly or indirectly, to the transmission of life and love."[17] What a profound challenge HIV/AIDS presents to the meaning and reality of sexual intercourse, now connecting death-dealing with life-and-love-giving. At the level of the human family, this new fact has great symbolic reverberations. At the level of individual couples, it raises the complex dilemmas we see in Lizzie Porter's case.

Authentic love necessarily desires the flourishing of life for self and the other. Surely, in some situations, the expression of love could risk losing one's life. Think of the martyrs past and present, for example, Archbishop Romero who risked (indeed gave up) his life in being faithful to the Gospel and in loving his people. What about our present topic, the sexual behavior of a couple when HIV/AIDS is present? Does this expression of love justify risking one's life, or are other means of loving possible? Can one ever risk another's life?

The Consistent Ethic of Life clearly emphasizes authentic love and the avoidance of unjustified risk. Any form of oppression, casual disregard for life, and rejection of available resources or of alternative expressions do not qualify as justifying risks. The deep desire to have a child might, though certainly such a decision needs careful discernment (as we saw in chapter 3). Although the Consistent Ethic when combined with a discerning methodology (chapter 2) recognizes the complexity of moral decisions, in this case there is a strong tilt in the direction of finding means of loving that avoid putting oneself or others at risk for HIV infection—and so promote life.

DEALINGS WITH HEALTH-CARE PROVIDERS

What about dealings with health-care providers: issues of privacy, confidentiality, truth-telling, and using experimental drugs? These first three topics, of course, have a long history in the discussions about patient-physician relationships. Foundational for honest and open communication, these essential elements nevertheless have been compromised in various ways.

We have already seen that in some situations a patient's disease must be reported, in some form, to public authorities. There may also be contact tracing. These requirements introduce limits and potential problems concerning privacy and confidentiality. Widespread use of technology has also increased the possibility of breaches of confidentiality, especially with access to information on computers.

In their discussion of confidentiality, Beauchamp and Childress describe the case of a physician on the staff of a New Jersey medical center. Within a few hours of being diagnosed as HIV-positive, "he received numerous phone calls of sympathy" from colleagues. Within a few days, he heard from patients, "and shortly thereafter his surgical privileges at the medical center were suspended and his practice ruined."[18]

Truth-telling raises its own set of dilemmas, often expressed in the tension between beneficence and autonomy. Beneficence is the principle that guides physicians to do the best for the patient. In some situations, for example, physicians have determined that full disclosure of the patient's condition may undermine the patient's desire to get well. Loss of hope may actually complicate the patient's condition.[19]

In recent years, patient advocates have challenged this form of beneficence, claiming that it has in fact slipped into paternalism. The physician decides what is best for the patient, without consultation. Advocates emphasize patient autonomy instead, stressing the importance of full knowledge and truly informed consent. This approach, they claim, better recognizes the dignity and freedom of the patient.[20]

An example of this tension is a physician who determines that a very distraught patient is HIV-positive. The physician concludes that informing the patient of her status at this time might push her over the edge—to very risky behavior or even suicide. For the good of the patient (beneficence), the doctor chooses not to tell the patient immediately but first attempts to help her with her depression.

Advocates of autonomy, emphasizing justice and moral relationship building, would argue that this paternalism in fact harms the patient, undermining her freedom and dignity. Rather she is to be informed and helped with her complete condition.

Autonomy, however, is not absolute. As Beauchamp and Childress argue (along with many others), autonomy is "one moral principle in a system of principles. . . . The human moral community, indeed morality itself, is rooted no less deeply in the three clusters of principles" of nonmalficence, beneficence, and justice.[21] In different situations, different principles are more important (as we have already seen, when justice or the common good outweighs individual freedom). Thus, the tensions remain.

The Consistent Ethic of Life recognizes these tensions. It has already been noted that the Consistent Ethic's roots include deep respect for the individual (human dignity) and for the community (common good). Holding these two together can clearly be challenging. Human dignity demands that the first move must always be toward confidentiality and truth-telling. But there may be times (as we have seen) that the common good outweighs individual rights.

Prudence, based on careful discernment, can direct which way the decision-maker ought to tilt in a particular situation—in order to promote the flourishing of life most fully. It is important to keep in mind not only the immediate case but also long-term consequences, for example, the damage done to patient-physician relationships in general if confidentiality and truth-telling are too easily violated.

The fourth issue of this fourth question, using experimental drugs and therapies, still needs to be considered. The issue, of course, surfaces in situations of need and perhaps desperation. The question may have been more pressing before the development of the effective anti-retroviral treatments. As people searched for something—anything—to save lives, some were willing to try experimental or even not-yet-approved drugs.

Now, at least for those with access to highly active antiretroviral therapy (HAART), the issue may be one of developing resistance and so needing to find new combinations that work.

The ethical issue focuses on risk: in the situation of HIV/AIDS, are there limits to the risks one may take in order to find some help? Because we are body people, we have a moral responsibility to care for our health. Ordinarily, this responsibility implies avoiding unnecessary or unjustified risks. Clearly, once a person is HIV-positive, conditions are greatly different, allowing for more risk-taking. Participating in trials of new drugs may even be considered a moral good, contributing to the common good through the development of new scientific knowledge. A sound patient-physician relationship can help the patient find responsible trials when necessary or possible.

Living with HIV and AIDS raises profound ethical dilemmas regarding one's relationships with other people. In this chapter we have considered a few of those situations and have seen how the Consistent Ethic of Life provides guidance for responding to these dilemmas. At times that guidance is very clear. At other times the complexity of the dilemmas demands a faith-filled prudence to discern the best choice in the concrete situation for true respect for life.

NOTES

1. J. McGowan, et al., "Risk Behavior for Transmission of Human Immunodeficiency Virus (HIV) among HIV-seropositive Individuals in an Urban Setting," *Clinical Infectious Diseases*, vol. 38, no. 1 (1 January 2004): 122–27. Also see articles cited in notes 2–7. An example of "unprotected sex" would be sexual intercourse without a condom. It must be noted that, while evidence shows that condoms have been very helpful in reducing HIV transmission, condom use does not guarantee "safe" sex.

2. Travis Porco, et al., "Decline in HIV Infectivity Following the Introduction of Highly Active Antiretroviral Therapy," *AIDS*, vol. 18, issue 1 (2 January 2004): 81–88.

3. Amy Rock Wohl, et al., "Recent Increase in High-Risk Sexual Behaviors among Sexually Active Men Who Have Sex with Men Living with AIDS in Los Angeles County," *Journal of Acquired Immune Deficiency Syndromes*, vol. 35, issue 2 (1 February 2004): 209–11.

4. Mark Clements, et al., "Modeling Trends in HIV Incidence among Homosexual Men in Australia," *Journal of Acquired Immune Deficiency Syndromes*, vol. 35, issue 4 (1 April 2004): 401–6.

5. Antonio Urbina and Kristina Jones, "Crystal Methamphetamine, Its Analogues, and HIV Infection: Medical and Psychiatric Aspects of a New Epidemic," *Clinical Infectious Diseases*, vol. 38, no. 6 (15 March 2004): 890–94.

6. Michael Carter, "Methamphetamine Use by New York Gay Men Risks Epidemic of Resistant HIV Warns Opinion Piece," *NAM*,www.aidsmap.com/en/news/73EEA791-D485-4E8C-80F7-9BA88BC17D52.asp (accessed 12 July 2004).

7. Cari L. Miller, et al., "The Future Face of Coinfection," *Journal of Acquired Immune Deficiency Syndromes*, vol. 36, Issue 2 (1 June 2004): 743–49.

8. Gillian Paterson, *Women in the Time of AIDS* (Maryknoll, N.Y.: Orbis Books, 1996), 1–3.

9. Paterson, *Women in the Time*, 3.

10. Paterson, *Women in the Time*, 4–10.

11. Dahleen Glanton, "Emerging Face of HIV," *Chicago Tribune*, 28 March 2004, 1.

12. Glanton, "Emerging Face," 17.

13. See John Mary Waliggo, "A Woman Confronts Social Stigma in Uganda," 48–57; Orlando Navarro Rojas, "Women and Children's Risks of Contracting HIV in Costa Rica," 135–41; and Laurenti Magesa, "Recognizing the Reality of African Religion in Tanzania," 76–84; in *Catholic Ethicists on HIV/AIDS Prevention*, ed. James F. Keenan, S.J. (New York: Continuum, 2002).

14. Amy L. Fairchild, James Colgrove, and Ronald Bayer, "The Myth of Exceptionalism," *Journal of Law, Medicine and Ethics*, vol. 31, no. 4 (Winter 2003).

15. Jeffrey P. Kahn, "HIV Test Reporting: Public Protection or Individual Punishment," (*Ethics Matters,* Center for Bioethics, University of Minnesota, 23 June 1998), *CNN*, www.cnn.com/Health/bioethics/archive.index.html (accessed 15 July 2004).

16. Glanton, "Emerging Face," 17; for a recent study of discordant couples, see R. E. Bunnell, et al., "Living with Discordance: Knowledge, Challenges, and Prevention Strategies of HIV-discordant couples in Uganda," *AIDS Care* 17, no. 8 (November 2005): 999–1012.

17. Pope John Paul II, "A Church Responding to the Sick and Poor," *Origins,* vol. 20, no. 15 (20 September 1990): 244.

18. Tom Beauchamp and James Childress, *Principles of Biomedical Ethics*, Fourth Edition (New York: Oxford University Press, 1994), 419. In the surgeon's situation, clearly there could be fear of the surgeon cutting himself during surgery and bleeding into the patient.

19. Beauchamp and Childress, *Principles,* 398–401.

20. Beauchamp and Childress, *Principles*, 120–88 and 259–325; also see Thomas Shannon, *Bioethics*, Third Edition (Mahwah, N.J.: Paulist Press, 1987), 5–16.

21. Beauchamp and Childress, *Principles*, 181.

Chapter Five

Ethics and the End of Life

HIV and AIDS raise ethical questions that extend throughout the life cycle and around the globe. In this chapter, we will consider the third cluster of these questions concerning the end of life. (1) How much pain must be endured? (2) What kinds of life-support treatment are appropriate? (3) Is there a limit to the resources to be used? (4) Is euthanasia or physician-assisted suicide a moral option?

Before considering these specific questions, let's take a careful look at the contemporary context of the topics and then the Church's long tradition about end-of-life issues, including its biblical roots.

While individuals and families and communities must face dying and death, in recent years certain people — their dying or their actions — have received front-page attention, for example, Karen Ann Quinlan, Nancy Cruzan, Terri Schiavo (all related to the question of withdrawal of life support systems), and Jack Kavorkian (for assisted suicide and euthanasia). Individual states' attempts to legalize assisted suicide and/or euthanasia also have received extensive media attention.

Proposals for euthanasia have a certain appeal, an appeal often emphasized by the media, because mercy killing *seems* to offer a solution to profound human fears: fear of being a burden on one's family; fear of unbearable pain; fear of having exhausted one's savings; and fear of prolonging death with tubes and machines.

Confusion often clouds the issue as well, especially when we face decisions about using life-support systems for ourselves or for relatives. When is there an obligation to use such technology, and when are we free not to use it? And how is this decision related to euthanasia?

The Catholic Church's long tradition about end-of-life treatments informs the perspectives of the Consistent Ethic and offers sound guidance in these complex issues.[1] Three major points emerge from the Scriptures: (1) life is a basic—but not absolute—good; (2) we are to be stewards of life, but we don't have complete control; and (3) we understand death in the context of belief in new life.

In the first creation story in Genesis, we hear of the goodness of all creation (1:31) and, in a special way, the sacredness of human life, for we are created in God's image (1:27). Human life, then, possesses a dignity, rooted in who we are rather than in what we do. Life is holy, deserving of respect and reverence. We know from our experience that life is the foundation for all other goods: friendship, love, prayer, and all the other ways we enjoy and serve God and neighbor.

Life, however, is not an absolute good. There is a greater good: our relationship with God. We would not, for example, destroy our relationship with God through sin in order to save our physical life. The powerful witness of the martyrs testifies to this truth. Jesus himself embodied this truth in his teaching and living, trusting in God and remaining faithful even to death on a cross (see Matthew 16:26 and Phil 2:5–11). Scripture makes it clear that life is a basic good but not an absolute one.[2]

Stewardship, our second major point, must be distinguished from unlimited and absolute control. Stewardship implies that we have the responsibility to care for something that is not totally our own possession. Control on the other hand claims an ultimate right to do whatever one wants. Beginning with Genesis, the Scriptures tell us again and again that we have stewardship over life but never absolute control. For life, as we have already seen, is a gift of God, to be respected and reverenced.

"To be stewards means to care for, to foster and nourish the gift of life—our own and that of others—so that our lives might flourish abundantly. Because we have been fashioned in the image of the Creator, we are, in a sense, 'co-creators.' "[3]

Jesus' whole life modeled the ideal of stewardship, creatively nourishing the gift of life (John 6:22–71) and humbly accepting that pain and suffering cannot always be eliminated (Mark 14:32–42).

The third point about choosing life that the Scriptures offer us is the conviction that death is not the final word. Death is not a transition from life to nothingness; rather, death marks the transformation to new and eternal life. This belief does not deny the reality of death, along with its suffering and separation. This belief promises that life is changed, not ended. We can look forward in hope to the fullness of life.

Our belief in everlasting life is rooted, of course, in the transforming experience of the resurrection of Jesus (see Luke 24:1–53 and John 20:1–21:25). This resurrection faith allows us to see that new life comes through death. We too trust in God's loving faithfulness.

How, then, do these three biblical insights—life is a basic good, we are stewards of life, and death is not the final word—enlighten the dilemmas of euthanasia, assisted suicide, and use of life-support systems?

The conviction that we are stewards of life grounds the opposition to euthanasia. We use our creativity to cure illness and promote wellness. As stewards, we respond with care and compassion to those who are suffering. Indeed, we have much to learn about better methods of pain control. We also acknowledge that we face limits, for not all pain can be eliminated and ultimately death cannot be avoided. Mercy killing, however, moves beyond stewardship. Euthanasia, even for compassionate reasons, implies that we have absolute control over life and so contradicts who we are as "co-creators."

Similarly, with assisted suicide, recognizing both the good gift of life and our responsibilities as stewards prohibits choosing suicide or helping someone else to end his or her life. Suicide, though rooted in frustration, pain, and despair, is an attempt to seize ultimate control over life. It too contradicts the fundamental reality of our lives.[4]

The decision for euthanasia or assisted suicide may seem to be very private, yet it has profound implications for society. Certainly the movement to legalize euthanasia and assisted suicide has brought the issues into the public forum. Public opinion polls often indicate widespread support. But is this support based on an emotional response or on careful and faithful reasoning? What impact on society would legalizing euthanasia have? Many are convinced that such a policy would further undermine reverence for life in our society, would reduce trust in the medical profession, and would put old and infirm people in very vulnerable positions. The public policy dimensions of the euthanasia issue are very serious and demand an intelligent, nuanced response that respects the dignity of all persons.[5]

The question of withdrawing or withholding life-support systems is distinct from—and yet often associated with—the question of euthanasia. Scriptural insights can be very helpful with this issue, even if they cannot give details. As good stewards, we believe that death is not the final word, that life is not an absolute good. Therefore, we do not have to keep someone alive "at all costs."

The Christian tradition has provided this guidance: ethically ordinary means must be used, ethically extraordinary means are optional. Ethically ordinary means are interventions that offer a reasonable hope of benefit and can be used without excessive expense, pain, or other inconvenience. Ethically extraordinary means do not offer reasonable hope of benefit or include excessive expense, pain, or other inconvenience. It is important to remember that "ordinary" and "extraordinary" refer not to the technology but to the treatment *in relation* to the condition of the patient; in other words, the proportion of benefit and burden the treatment provides the patient.[6]

Many people remember when Cardinal Bernardin decided to stop the treatment for his cancer. The treatment had become "ethically extraordinary." He did not kill himself by this choice but did stop efforts that prolonged his dying. He allowed death to occur. Many of us know of similar cases in our own families.

In some situations, removing life-support systems, including feeding tubes, is morally the same kind of action. We are not starving a person to death but choosing to stop efforts that attempted to avoid death. Providing medical nourishment through a feeding tube is something very different from giving a person a bowl of soup with a spoon, and so this procedure can also become an "ethically extraordinary" means of life support. To stop it is not to cause death but to allow death to occur. The cause, the condition that keeps the person from swallowing enough food to stay alive, is already present in the person, just like Cardinal Bernardin's cancer. (For cautions, see "Nutrition and Hydration: Moral and Pastoral Reflections" by the U.S. Bishops' Committee for Pro-Life Activities.)[7]

Within the Catholic Church however, debate still surrounds this question of withdrawing artificial nutrition and hydration. While one position holds that medical nourishment must be provided in almost all cases, another position asks what possibility the sick person has for pursuing life's purposes—happiness, fulfillment, and love of God and neighbor—when discerning whether the life support can be removed. If a fatal disease or condition is present and if life-prolonging efforts would be useless or a severe burden in pursuing life's purposes, then we can withdraw the feeding tubes and allow the person to die as a result of the fatal disease or condition. This position strongly opposes euthanasia, affirms the individual's right to be the primary decision-maker, and stresses the moral distinction between allowing a person to die and killing that person.[8] Two other factors that must be included in deciding what to do are extensive consultation with medical experts and appropriate use of scarce medical resources.

We do not have to do everything possible in every situation to keep a person alive. We can allow the individual to die, entrusting that person to our loving and faithful God. Focusing on the distinction between "allowing to die" and "killing" leads to clarity about what is really happening and emphasizes the difference between a deep respect for life and the desire to control life and death.[9]

Euthanasia evokes powerful emotions and may seem to be merciful when sincere people desire to help suffering people. Our Scriptures, however, point in a different direction. We can allow someone to die, but we must never kill. And always we must be present with care and compassion.

Let's see, then, how this tradition helps in answering the questions of this chapter related to HIV/AIDS.

PAIN

How much pain must be endured? As little as possible, of course, but sometimes that may be substantial. Two aspects of this question deserve careful consideration: the possible implication that serious suffering may open the door to euthanasia or assisted suicide and the theory and practice of pain management.

Euthanasia

Pain and other forms of suffering certainly challenge individuals, their families, and communities. HIV/AIDS, of course, challenges entire nations and the global community. Such suffering also challenges philosophical and theological perspectives that attempt to shed light on this common human experience.

From "common sense" and some philosophical approaches, many persons have concluded that such pain and suffering undermine human dignity and so must be resisted—sometimes at all costs. A person ought not to be forced to endure pain beyond a certain tolerable level and must be free to control one's destiny. Such control can take the ultimate form of ending one's life in order to stop the pain. Thus the movements to legalize assisted suicide and euthanasia.

A famous case in the 1980s stands as a symbol of this conviction. An anonymous article published in the highly respected *Journal of the American Medical Association* (*JAMA*) described a gynecology resident's decision to give a young cancer patient a lethal dose of morphine. "It's Over, Debbie" gives a first-person account of the event. The doctor describes the whole experience in a very factual tone: being upset with the call in the middle of the night, going to the oncology unit and meeting a previously unknown twenty-year-old patient, reviewing her condition, calling the situation "a gallows scene, a cruel mockery of her youth and unfulfilled potential,"[10] and hearing her only words of "Let's get this over with." So the doctor asks the nurse for morphine and injects the patient with enough "to do the job."[11] It does, and she dies. "It's over, Debbie."

The article "provoked a storm of outrage"[12] but also led to serious and open discussion about euthanasia and assisted suicide. On the outrage side: four physicians (Willard Gaylin, Leon Kass, Edmund Pellegrino, and Mark Siegler) wrote a stinging critique of "It's Over, Debbie," both as an article (that was published by *JAMA* without editorial comment) and as an action (murder). They go on to describe the action as "a profound violation of the deepest meaning of the medical vocation."[13]

Kass went on to write his own article, a long, probing essay.[14] In it he spells out his reasons for claiming that euthanasia by physicians "is a bad idea whose time must not come—not now, not ever."[15] He addresses this topic in the larger context of medicine as "an inherently ethical activity."[16] Kass states that the central core of medicine is to heal, to make whole. Euthanasia contradicts this central core. "To say it plainly, to bring nothingness is incompatible with serving wholeness: one cannot heal—or comfort—by making nil. The healer cannot annihilate if he is truly to heal. The boundary condition, 'No deadly drugs,' flows directly from the center, 'Make whole.' "[17]

On the other side: a year after "It's Over, Debbie," a number of physicians from leading medical centers published an article in the *New England Journal of Medicine* that supported physician-assisted suicide.[18] Concerning pain, the authors are very clear: "The hopelessly ill patient must have whatever is necessary to control pain. . . . Narcotics or other pain medication should be given in whatever dose and by whatever route is necessary for relief. . . . To allow a patient to experience unbearable pain or suffering is unethical medical practice."[19]

Moving from pain relief to assisted suicide, the physicians acknowledge that proper pain relief occasionally fails. In such situations some patients ask for help in ending their lives. (Note: in a suicide, the final act is performed by the patient, that is, by swallowing a sufficient number of sleeping pills.) The authors also acknowledge that some physicians do indeed assist in such suicides, "believing it to be the last act in a continuum of care provided for the helplessly ill patient."[20] After discussing some related questions and concerns, the physicians conclude "that it is not immoral for a physician to assist in the rational suicide of a terminally ill person."[21]

They hesitate, however, concerning euthanasia. (Note: in euthanasia, the physician performs a medical procedure that causes death directly, e.g., a lethal injection.) The authors note that many physicians oppose euthanasia because of moral or religious reasons, because they believe it does not fit a physician's role, or because they fear it could lead to involuntary euthanasia. Finally, the authors state "the prospect of criminal prosecution deters even the hardiest advocates of euthanasia among physicians."[22]

Several months earlier, the executive editor of the *New England Journal of Medicine*, Marcia Angell, succinctly summarized the debate about euthanasia in its early stages. "For many, the beginning of a debate about euthanasia is ominous—a step down a slippery slope leading to widespread disregard for the value of human life. For others, it signifies an opportunity to deal more humanely and rationally with prolonged meaningless suffering."[23]

Several years later the same journal published "Death and Dignity: A Case of Individualized Decision Making" by Timothy Quill, M.D. In it he reports "how he had given instructions and provided adequate supplies of barbituates so that Diane, a patient he had known and treated for years who was now dying of cervical cancer, could and did end her life."[24] John Paris reports that there was little negative reaction to Quill's action but rather approval, because, it seems, Quill provided "comprehensive medical care, with deep concern for the patient's well being and respect for her choices."[25]

These early articles highlight many of the key aspects of the issue that have continued to be debated.

The Consistent Ethic of Life follows the long Catholic tradition in affirming that pain is to be resisted, even with strong medications that may indirectly shorten life. However, pain is not considered a sufficient (proportionate) reason to cause death.[26] Causing death, even though for merciful reasons, contradicts the nature of human beings as "co-creators," as stewards of life who do not have absolute control over life and death.

Pain Management

The second dimension of this first question about pain, then, is the theory and practice of pain management. Studies often show that physicians are not successful in managing their patients' pain.[27] On the other hand, the Hospice movement has taken pain management and palliative care very seriously and is quite successful in most cases.[28] Clearly, such insights need to be spread throughout the practice of medicine.

Pain and suffering raise not only ethical and medical questions but also theological ones. Before concluding this first question, it seems right to consider briefly the ancient question of suffering and its meaning. The world's religions have grappled with this mystery. Some responses in the Christian tradition, while popular, may also be problematic. Let this quotation from the Vatican's *Declaration on Euthanasia* be an example.

"According to Christian teaching, however, suffering, especially suffering during the last moments of life, has a special place in God's saving plan; it is, in fact, a sharing in Christ's Passion and a union with the redeeming sacrifice which he offered in obedience to the father's will. Therefore, one must not be surprised if some Christians prefer to moderate their use of painkillers, in order to accept voluntarily at least a part of their sufferings and, thus, associate themselves in a conscious way with the sufferings of Christ crucified."[29]

This view, rooted in particular understandings of atonement and sacrifice, raises questions about how the God of Jesus could will suffering and how reducing painkillers could be pleasing to God.[30]

Another Christian perspective, grounded in John's Gospel and in the letters to the Colossians and to the Ephesians and developed throughout the tradition by such scholars as John Duns Scotus and Karl Rahner, interprets suffering differently because it interprets the purpose of Jesus's life differently. Jesus is not an afterthought to original sin; he was not sent to suffer to make up for sin. Rather, Jesus is God's first thought, the culmination of God's self-communication, the purpose of all creation.[31]

Suffering, then, is seen as a part of life, not something willed by God. Christians respond to suffering by following Jesus's own pattern: resisting evil, working to overcome it, and always trusting in a present and faithful God.[32] Regarding HIV/AIDS in particular, this view affirms that such suffering is not a punishment sent by God (as some religious leaders proclaim). Rather, followers of Jesus must do their best to promote treatment, prevention, healing—and comfort and presence when medicine fails.

LIFE-SUPPORT TREATMENT

What kinds of life-support treatment are appropriate? As with so many of the questions in this book, the response depends on the social setting, with resources ranging from the newest and best treatments to almost nothing. This latter situation again raises the justice issue regarding economic and political structures (to be considered in more detail in the next two chapters). In this chapter, it is sufficient to concentrate on more personal issues.

The review of the Catholic tradition's teaching about end-of-life topics highlights both the responsibility to care for one's health and life and the freedom to stop treatment in some situations. Accordingly, an HIV-positive person has the moral responsibility to seek treatment, making use of medications that can help preserve life. Such a response is important for the individual and for those who are related to the person, especially children. Highly active antiretroviral therapy (HAART) can rightly be considered life-support treatment.

For those for whom such treatment fails or is not available, then the question of life support (understood in more traditional terms) enters the picture. As with other diseases and life-threatening situations, the tradition offers sound guidance. When the burden of pursuing life's purposes outweighs the benefits, then treatment can be stopped. But caregivers must always try to provide as much palliative care as possible to reduce pain and keep the individual as comfortable as possible. Compassionate presence is always important. As we saw in the first question, pain control and compassionate care do not include killing.

One more aspect of this situation deserves careful attention. There is now the rather curious situation in the United States where health-care providers are forced to sue families in order to stop treatment of some patients. The health-care providers have determined that such treatment is futile, offering no reasonable hope and only using up scarce resources. The families are demanding that "everything be done" to keep their loved one alive.[33]

This dilemma, perhaps partly rooted in medicine's past practices of overly aggressive treatment, raises concerns for justice in the use of scarce resources. The Catholic tradition, as we have seen, allows people to stop treatment but has not said people *must* stop treatment. Nevertheless, a careful appreciation of the social teachings with emphasis on the common good may well point in this direction, especially when the best medical judgment concludes that the treatment is futile. The next question clearly follows from this dilemma.

RESOURCES

Is there a limit to the resources to be used? What a delicate and complex question! Clearly the answer must be Yes—for we live in a world of limited resources. The question, of course, is how to determine this limit in a fair and accurate way. Again, this point spills over into the next two chapters. Focusing on the personal dimension here returns us to the previous question. Individuals (and those who represent them) can respect the reality of the world's limited resources by deliberately choosing to forego all futile treatment and even all treatment in which the burdens outweigh the benefits.

A prominent U.S. Scripture scholar even went beyond this. Aware of the great difference in medical care available to people in resource-rich countries and to those in resource-poor countries and desiring to express his solidarity with the poor, this scholar expressed in his living will (for more on advance directives, please see appendix II) his desire to receive only that treatment possible for the poor in the developing world. After suffering a severe stroke, he was simply given comfort care before he died.

Few will follow the depths of commitment to the poor expressed in this example. Still, until the massive split between rich and poor is overcome, such selfless awareness and sensitivity is a remarkable response to the question of determining a fair allocation of scarce resources. On the other hand, hundreds of millions of people in our world face the same situation but without any choice. Without many resources, death happens.

This reality led philosopher John Kavanaugh, S.J., while commenting on John Paul II's remarks on feeding tubes, to state: "The pope's talk is as much a challenge to our health-care system and the inequities in the world as it is to our treatment of patients. Why can we not see that? Perhaps the answer lies in the strange phenomenon that a small percentage of the world's privileged can worry whether they must use every technology to feed themselves while millions do not even have bread and clean water."[34]

EUTHANASIA OR PHYSICIAN-ASSISTED SUICIDE

Is euthanasia or physician-assisted suicide a moral option? The emotional pull toward this option is extremely strong. Wouldn't it be the merciful action to take in order to end suffering? Is there really any difference between a lethal injection and the withdrawal of life support? Indeed, isn't the injection better since it shortens the suffering-and-dying process?

We have already seen both sides of these questions. Still, it is essential to appreciate the strength of the emotional appeal and the other fears that fuel the push toward euthanasia and physician-assisted suicide. These emotional motives can easily seem to trump careful moral reasoning.[35]

The heart of the Catholic tradition's position, and so the heart of the Consistent Ethic of Life, is the faith conviction that human beings are creatures and stewards, images of God who have responsibility to care for the gift of life. This faith-inspired understanding of the reality of life leads to the rejection of euthanasia and physician-assisted suicide as contradictions of what it means to be truly human. Euthanasia undermines rather than promotes human flourishing.[36] Even the positive motivation of mercy is not sufficient to outweigh the evil of killing. Other options are possible. A real and important distinction remains between killing and allowing to die—not ultimately for the patient but for the person who performs the action.

In a pluralistic society, it is necessary to look for additional reasons than just faith-based ones. We have already considered some of these in the first question of this chapter. Euthanasia and physician assisted suicide would violate the meaning of the medical vocation, would undermine trust in physicians ("When does my doctor become my executioner?"), and would put vulnerable people at greater risk (the old and infirm, and women in general—because they live longer than men, have fewer resources, and have long been socialized to "sacrifice themselves" for others).[37]

When medicine fails, the Consistent Ethic of Life urges compassionate care and loving presence, not mercy killing.

NOTES

1. John Paris and Richard McCormick, "The Catholic Tradition on the Use of Nutrition and Fluids," *America,* vol. 156, no. 17 (2 May 1987): 356–61; Ronald Hamel and Michael Panicola, "Must We Preserve Life?" *America*, vol. 190, no. 14 (19–26 April 2004): 6–13.

2. Hamel and Panicola, "Must We Preserve Life?" 7.

3. The Ohio Catholic Conference of Bishops, *Hopes and Fears: Pastoral Reflections on Death* (Columbus: Catholic Conference of Ohio, 1993), 2.

4. Ohio Catholic Conference, *Hopes and Fears*, 4; such a judgment, of course, is about the act, not the person, who may feel that he or she has no other choice.

5. Joseph Cardinal Bernardin, "Letter to the Supreme Court," in *A Moral Vision for America,* ed. John P. Langan, S.J. (Washington, D.C.: Georgetown University Press, 1998), 129–30.

6. Sacred Congregation for the Doctrine of the Faith, *Declaration on Euthanasia*, 1980; can be found in *Mercy or Murder?* ed. Kenneth R. Overberg, S.J. (Kansas City: Sheed & Ward, 1993), 140–50 at 146–48.

7. USCCB Committee on Pro-Life Activities, *Nutrition and Hydration: Moral and Pastoral Reflections* (Washington, D.C.: USCCB Publications Service, 1992).

8. John Paris, S.J., "Hugh Finn's 'Right to Die,'" *America,* vol. 179, no. 13 (31 October 1998): 13–15. See also Richard A. McCormick, S.J., "'Moral Considerations' Ill Considered," *America,* vol. 166, no. 9 (14 March 1992): 210–14; also found in *Mercy or Murder?* 252–61.

9. Richard A. McCormick, S.J., "*Vive la Difference!* Killing and Allowing to Die," *America,* vol. 177, no. 18 (6 December 1997): 6–12.

10. Anonymous, "It's Over, Debbie," in *Mercy or Murder?* 57.

11. Anonymous, "It's Over, Debbie," in *Mercy or Murder?* 57.

12. John Paris, S.J., "Active Euthanasia," *Theological Studies,* 53, no. 1 (March 1992): 113–26; also in *Mercy or Murder?* 3–20 at 9.

13. Willard Gaylin, M.D., Leon R. Kass, M.D., Edmund D. Pellegrino, M.D., and Mark Siegler, M.D., "Doctors Must Not Kill," *Journal of the American Medical Association,* 259, no. 14 (8 April 1988): 2139–40; also in *Mercy or Murder?* 125–29 at 126.

14. Leon R. Kass, M.D., "Neither for Love nor Money: Why Doctors Must Not Kill," *Public Interest,* vol. 94 (Winter 1989): 25–46; also in *Mercy or Murder?* 97–124.

15. Kass, M.D., "Neither for Love nor Money," 98.

16. Kass, M.D., "Neither for Love nor Money," 101.

17. Kass, M.D., "Neither for Love nor Money," 117.

18. Sidney H. Wanzer, M.D., Daniel D. Federman, M.D., S. James Adelstein, M.D., Christine K. Cassel, M.D., Edwin H. Cassem, M.D., Ronald E. Cranford, M.D., Edward W. Hook, M.D., et al, "The Physician's Responsibility Toward Hopelessly Ill Patients: A Second Look," *New England Journal of Medicine,* 320, no. 13 (30 March 1989): 844–49; also in *Mercy or Murder?* 38–55.

19. Wanzer, et al., "Physician's Responsibility," 46–47.

20. Wanzer, et al., "Physician's Responsibility," 49.

21. Wanzer, et al., "Physician's Responsibility," 51.

22. Wanzer, et al., "Physician's Responsibility," 53.

23. Marcia Angell, M.D., "Euthanasia," *New England Journal of Medicine,* 319, no. 20 (17 November 1988): 1348–50; also in *Mercy or Murder?* 32–37 at 32.

24. Paris, S.J., "Active Euthanasia," 11.

25. Paris, S.J., "Active Euthanasia," 11.

26. Congregation for the Doctrine of the Faith, *Euthanasia,* 145–47.

27. Wanzer, et al., "Physician's Responsibility," 45–46.

28. Walter B. Forman, ed., *Hospice and Palliative Care* (Sudbury, Mass.: Jones and Bartlett, 2003), 143–59; Carolyn Jaffe and Carol H. Ehrlich, *All Kinds of Love* (Amityville, N.Y.: Baywood Publishers, 1997), 197–211 and 215–43; it is also important to note the value of using palliative care principles as complementary care to other treatment throughout the course of HIV infection.

29. Congregation for the Doctrine of the Faith, *Euthanasia*, 145.

30. Kenneth R. Overberg, S.J., *Into the Abyss of Suffering* (Cincinnati: St. Anthony Messenger Press, 2003), 51–71. See also appendix I.

31. Overberg, S.J., *Into the Abyss*, 73–93.

32. Overberg, S.J., *Into the Abyss*, 95–119.

33. James F. Drane and John L. Coulehan, "The Concept of Futility: Patients Do Not Have a Right to Demand Medically Useless Treatment," *Health Progress*, 74, no. 10 (December 1993): 28–32; also see Robert M. Veatch and Carol Mason Spicer, "Futile Care: Physicians Should Not Be Allowed to Refuse to Treat," *Health Progress*, 74, no. 10 (December 1993): 22–27.

34. John F. Kavanaugh, S.J., "Artificial Feeding," *America*, vol. 190, no. 20 (21–28 June 2004): 7.

35. Peter A. Singer, M.D., and Mark Siegler, M.D., "Euthanasia—A Critique," *New England Journal of Medicine*, 322, no. 26 (28 June 1990): 1881–83; also in *Mercy or Murder?* 130–39 at 133.

36. Bernardin, "Euthanasia in the Catholic Tradition," in *A Moral Vision* 126–28.

37. Gaylin, M.D., Kass, M.D., Pellegrino, M.D., Siegler, M.D., "Doctors Must Not Kill," 128; see also Margaret A. Farley, "Issues in Contemporary Christian Ethics: The Choice of Death in a Medical Context," *Moral Issues and Christian Response*, sixth edition (Fort Worth Tex.:Harcourt Brace, 1998), 427–28.

Chapter Six

Ethics and Society

HIV and AIDS raise ethical questions that extend throughout the life cycle and around the globe. In this chapter, we will consider the fourth cluster of these questions concerning society's policies and responsibilities. (1) Does the common good of society demand testing for HIV, and who will be tested: health-care personnel, those with high-risk behaviors, those who apply for marriage licenses, those convicted of crimes, or everyone? (2) What are societies' responsibilities concerning costs related to HIV/AIDS? (3) Is there a moral obligation concerning educational programs in light of the growing epidemic? (4) Should programs that promote the use of condoms or needle exchange be supported? (5) What about the effects of prejudice against HIV-infected persons and their families and friends in housing, parishes, employment, insurance, and medical treatment?

As noted in chapter 2, the Consistent Ethic of Life was developed to help shape public policy. Economic structures and political decisions profoundly help or hinder the flourishing of all life. Our list of questions concerning society's responsibilities points to crucial and often ambiguous issues with significant moral implications. The Consistent Ethic of Life balances its concern for the individual person with its emphasis on the common good. Human dignity and solidarity, then, provide the insights for creatively resolving the tensions between individual and society.

Many of the questions in our list date back to the early years of the epidemic. Ignorance, fear, and prejudice often led to extreme policy recommendations and even practices. Advocacy groups responded aggressively, working to protect privacy and freedom.[1]

As with most of the issues related to HIV/AIDS, cultural context plays a major role in framing these questions and responding to them. Prejudice and stigmatization, for example, will be experienced in very different ways in India or the United States.[2] Keeping those kinds of differences in mind, let's look at this cluster of questions in more detail.

TESTING FOR HIV

Does the common good of society demand testing for HIV, and who will be tested: health-care personnel, those with high-risk behaviors, those who apply for marriage licenses, those convicted of crimes, or everyone? The issue of testing was partially included in chapter 4, in the discussion of the second question on partner notification. Society's responsibility to respond to the epidemic along with epidemiologists' emphasis on the importance of testing clashed with individuals' claim for privacy in the face of various forms of prejudice.

While some nations refused (and still refuse) to acknowledge the presence of HIV/AIDS in their countries, others moved to the other extreme, even calling for quarantine.[3] Most societies ended up somewhere between these extremes, though testing has been limited in many developing countries by lack of resources.

Three types of testing have evolved: voluntary, routine, and mandatory. In voluntary testing for HIV, an individual chooses to have the test and so seeks out a testing center. Counseling is usually provided before and after the test. This counseling takes time, is designed to help the individual reduce risk, and may lead to treatment, follow-up counseling, and support groups. In routine testing, the HIV test is offered to people as part of another health-care service, that is, preparing for childbirth. In such situations, the individual's consent is still required, but risk reduction counseling and partner notification may be abbreviated or omitted. Mandatory testing comes in several forms: (1) the HIV test is required for a certain job or action; the individual can refuse the test but also then is prevented from getting the job or doing the action; (2) the HIV test is legally required; consent is not required; if the individual refuses the test, it will still be done; and (3) the HIV test is performed without the individual's knowledge; rarely in such situations is there either counseling or confidentiality.

In the United States the discussion about testing developed along two predictable positions: one emphasized public health and policies of control, the other confidentiality and individual rights. Writing at the end of the first decade of the epidemic, Ronald Bayer described the division between conservative political movements that urged broad legal provisions to control the spread of HIV/AIDS and liberal groups that pressed for HIV exceptionalism, freeing this epidemic from standard medical practices, including treating HIV tests like other blood tests, especially for pregnant women and newborn children.[4]

Bayer added:

> Inevitably, public health officials must contend with a range of extraprofessional considerations, including the prevailing political climate and the unique social forces brought into play by a particular public health challenge. In the first years of the AIDS epidemic, U.S. officials had no alternative but to negotiate the course of AIDS policy with representatives of a well-organized gay community and their allies in the medical and political establishments. In this process, many of the traditional practices of public health that might have been brought to bear were dismissed as inappropriate. As the first decade of the epidemic came to an end, public health officials began to reassert their professional dominance over the policy-making process and in so doing began to rediscover the relevance of their own professional traditions to the control of AIDS.[5]

Recognizing the tension between the two perspectives led Marcia Angell, then executive director of *The New England Journal of Medicine*, to recommend a dual approach to the epidemic.[6] This approach would distinguish social problems (for example, prejudice in housing or insurance) from epidemiologic problems. She was convinced that addressing social and economic concerns would allow greater attention to the medical problems.

> Concerning testing and related issues, Angell recommended the following: I believe that, on balance, systematic tracing and notification of the sexual partners of HIV-infected persons and screening of pregnant women, newborns, hospitalized patients, and health care professionals are warranted. These populations are, after all, relatively accessible to the health care system and at some special risk. Attempting to screen the

entire population would simply be impractical; on the other hand, target-
ing only high-risk groups would be unworkable, in part because it would
entail making distinctions that are often impossible as well as invidious.
With any increase in screening, however, the specter of discrimination
arises once a person is known to be infected. Only if such discrimination,
at least in its more tangible expressions, is countered by statute and if
those with HIV infection are assured of receiving all the medical care
they need, can we pursue the basic elements of infection control more
resolutely and so spare others the tragedy of this disease.7

Challenges to Angell's proposals came quickly from June Osborn
and David Rogers of the National Commission on AIDS.[8] They pointed
out that scientists working on HIV/AIDS did not support the testing of
all patients and all doctors and nurses and that resistance to testing pregnant women was based on a two-year study that concluded that testing
would be counterproductive.[9]

Rogers and Osborn acknowledged that Angell's dual approach
sounded reasonable, but ultimately would fail. They stressed four
points: (1) that tough laws would not eliminate discrimination; (2) that
basic health-care services should be made available to all, before special financing for an AIDS program; (3) that explicit, culturally appropriate education would reach more people with better results than routine testing, though voluntary testing needed to be promoted
aggressively; and (4) that the best way to protect patients is to insist on
universal precautions by health-care professionals.[10]

Before considering how this debate continues in the present, let's
look at what the Catholic bishops of the United States were saying
about testing shortly before the publication of the remarks of Bayer, Angell, and Rogers and Osborn. In their two major statements, *The Many
Faces of AIDS: A Gospel Response* and *Called to Compassion and Responsibility: A Response to the HIV/AIDS Crisis*, the bishops recognized the value of some testing programs but rejected universal mandatory testing.[11]

The bishops state that voluntary testing is needed as a matter of public policy.

These voluntary programs should always guarantee anonymity and
should be preceded and followed by necessary counseling for individuals
diagnosed as HIV-positive or negative. Counseling should supply infor-

mation about the disease, the moral aspects involved, immediate emotional support, and information about resources for continuing emotional and spiritual support. It should also underscore, sensitively but forthrightly, the grave moral responsibility of individuals with HIV to inform others who are at risk because of their condition.[12]

Reflecting the Catholic social teaching's emphasis on both human dignity and solidarity, the bishops attempt to balance individual and community rights and interests. "Two objectives are fundamental to any adequate understanding of the common good: first, preserving and protecting human dignity while guaranteeing the rights of all; second, caring for all who need help and cannot help themselves."[13] Applied to testing this means that people be informed when they are tested, for example when donating blood, that they receive the results, and that counseling be available.

The bishops then go on to discuss when the common good can outweigh the presumption in favor of confidentiality. They mention the need to prevent the infection of others and the need to provide medical care to the infected person.[14]

The success, expanding availability of, and access to more antiretroviral therapies has increased the demand for testing, both for treatment and prevention reasons. HIV testing is the entry point to treatment, care, and prevention services. If a person tests positive for HIV, this person can begin the process of treatment. An HIV-infected pregnant woman can start an antiretroviral regimen to prevent transmission to her baby. When combined with effective counseling, testing supports individuals and couples in their efforts to reduce or eliminate risky behaviors (if negative) and to prevent further transmission of the infection (if positive). However, the contemporary debate about testing repeats a number of the main themes we have already considered. In addition, as the epidemic continues unabated, there are movements around the world to require testing for various groups including immigrants and criminals.

In the United States, for example, mandatory testing is required for all applicants to the Armed Forces, Job Corps, and Peace Corps; for overseas State Department positions; for federal prisoners; and for people seeking legal residency (green card). Resistance, however, remains strong. Those who promote voluntary or routine testing claim that the advantages of mandatory testing sound good but are not found in practice. In fact, mandatory testing ends up being counterproductive, leading people to avoid medical treatment because of fear of stigma and discrimination. Mandatory testing does not prevent risky behavior. Treatment is often not available to those who test positive. In fact, these opponents claim, mandatory testing leads to negative public health outcomes.[15]

Concern for human rights violations is common. Two different policies in different parts of the world have led to similar resistance and so serve as good examples. In Peru there was a movement to legalize mandatory HIV testing for all pregnant women. The newspaper *El Comercio* praised the availability of counseling and testing, as long as the testing was voluntary. The paper indicated that international "research suggests that mandatory HIV testing undermines human rights and is potentially detrimental for public health."[16]

El Comercio adds:

> Mandatory HIV testing threatens to create situations that favor a range of human rights violations. The rights under threat include the rights to nondiscrimination and bodily integrity, the right to be free from violence, and the right to the highest attainable standard of health. This is particularly true for many women, who already find their human rights may be threatened or violated on a daily basis because of their sex. In 1998, the United Nations issued guidelines on HIV/AIDS and human rights that strongly support voluntary—not mandatory—HIV testing as a critical part of the fight against AIDS. A legislative reform in favor of mandatory HIV testing for pregnant women flies in the face of established human rights standards on HIV/AIDS. Those who promote mandatory testing seem to think that forcing pregnant women to be tested for HIV may benefit women, at least when treatment is broadly available. This argument does not account for the potential adverse public health effects of mandatory testing. It also ignores Peru's obligation in terms of human rights.[17]

A proposal for mandatory HIV testing before marriage in India produced similar resistance. Included among the reasons given for opposing the proposal were (1) mandatory testing drives the epidemic underground by deterring people from getting information and making use of services; (2) it violates a person's right to consent and confidentiality; (3) it does not address infection after marriage from unfaithful husbands; (4) it does not deal with false positives; and (5) it would be very costly.[18]

The author points out that many states in the United States considered mandatory testing, but only Illinois and Louisiana implemented the law—only to repeal it later.

Such opposition to mandatory testing reflects the positions of such groups as the World Health Organization and the Joint United Nations Programme on HIV and AIDS (UNAIDS). Opponents of mandatory testing continue to emphasize the "3Cs": confidentiality, counseling, and consent. The following, for example, summarizes the position of UNAIDS.

UNAIDS promotes expanded access to both client-initiated and provider-initiated voluntary, confidential HIV testing, conducted with informed consent and accompanied by counselling for both HIV-positive and HIV-negative individuals. With respect to provider-initiated testing, in all settings, individuals retain the right to refuse testing, e.g. to 'opt out' of a routine offer of testing. All testing needs to be accompanied by referral to medical and psychosocial services for those who receive a positive test result, and by community education and legal and policy reform to counter stigma and discrimination.[19]

Perhaps the most controversial topic is the testing of prisoners. Even in countries where human rights are recognized and protected, prisoners can too easily suffer abuse. So there is much concern about mandatory testing. On the other hand, the statistics and prison realities are staggering: more than two million people are incarcerated in the United States. Among these people the prevalence rate of HIV/AIDS is much higher than the general public. While a majority of HIV-positive prisoners were infected before entering prison, high-risk activities—injecting drug use, sexual activity, even tattooing—contribute to HIV transmission in prisons.[20] What, then, ought prison administrators do about testing and treatment?

In the United States, there are different answers to this question. All federal prisoners face mandatory testing, at least before they are discharged. A number of states have mandatory testing in their prisons, sometimes segregating those prisoners who are HIV-positive or at least those who have developed HIV-related diseases. Some states that once had mandatory testing or separate AIDS housing have discontinued these practices because of cost and inefficiency.

Opponents of these practices stress consent and confidentiality, appealing to the human rights of prisoners. Opponents also cite international policies from UNAIDS and the World Health Organization that urge the prohibition of mandatory testing, calling it unethical and ineffective.[21]

The International Guidelines on HIV/AIDS and Human Rights (published by UNAIDS and the UN High Commissioner for Human Rights) offer alternate measures to reduce the spread of HIV in prisons.

> Prison authorities should take all necessary measures, including adequate staffing, effective surveillance and appropriate disciplinary measures, to protect prisoners from rape, sexual violence and coercion. Prison authorities should also provide prisoners (and prison staff, as appropriate), with access to HIV-related prevention information, education, voluntary testing and counseling, means of prevention (condoms, bleach and clean injection equipment), treatment and care and voluntary participation in HIV-related clinical trials, as well as ensure confidentiality.[22]

The perceived tension between individual rights and the common good emerges clearly even from this brief description. Separating HIV-positive prisoners from other prisoners would seem to be an effective means for reducing the spread of HIV. (These are, of course, the same problems with any testing program: the window period during which recently infected persons do not test positive, false positives in the testing process, and cost.) However, separating prisoners, as with quarantine in the general public, may in the long run undermine the common good by limiting fundamental human rights. As suggested by the International Guidelines, there are other means available, although experience shows that these means require resources and commitment to be fully implemented.

The Catholic bishops' conference of the United States has not issued a detailed statement on AIDS since *Called to Compassion and Responsibility* in 1989. In that document the bishops opposed universal mandatory testing but did allow for mandatory testing in some limited situations. Indeed, some dioceses require HIV testing before a person can be admitted to the seminary (the type of mandatory testing that can be refused—along with one's desired goal, in this case preparation for ordination). In other parts of the world, Catholic bishops have supported mandatory testing in other situations, such as before marriage.

The Consistent Ethic of Life, with its roots in the social teachings, combines the individual and the common good, human dignity and solidarity. Prudential weighing of concrete situations and careful attention to facts may still lead to different conclusions about whether mandatory testing is justified in specific cases. Long-term consequences are particularly difficult to discuss. The experience and insight of the international groups (WHO and UNAIDS, for example) can be especially helpful for such discernment.

COSTS

What are societies' responsibilities concerning costs related to HIV/AIDS? Many of the nations most severely impacted by HIV and AIDS have already been overwhelmed by poverty, disease, violence, and war. Not surprisingly then, these nations have few resources to respond to their peoples' needs in confronting the epidemic. Clearly, some form of international aid is necessary if there is to be any hope of helping the millions of people in these countries.

Four examples of programs providing such aid are (1) The Global Fund to Fight AIDS, Tuberculosis and Malaria (GFATM); (2) WHO's 3X5 program; (3) the Clinton Foundation; and (4) the President's Emergency Plan for AIDS Relief (PEPFAR) of President Bush.

Global Fund to Fight AIDS, Tuberculosis and Malaria

In 2001, the Secretary General of the United Nations, Kofi Annan, proposed a global fund to assist resource-limited countries. The Global Fund to Fight AIDS, Tuberculosis and Malaria was created in 2002 to raise funds from governments, businesses, and individuals in order to support projects fighting these diseases.

Around fifty countries have offered support for the GFATM, and more than 120 countries have received or will receive funds. In 2005, 61 percent of the money was given to African countries. These funds must be requested by the individual country or organization. Over half of the funds were for AIDS projects in 2005, but this percentage depends on the requests and approvals. Each country must form a "Country Coordinating Mechanism" to oversee applications and to monitor implementation.

As of 2005 more than $6 billion had been pledged and more than $3.6 billion paid by the donors. Already by 2005, however, current projects were underfunded, and this serious funding gap threatened the continuation of these projects and, of course, did not allow for new ones.

Wealthy countries may be hesitant to fill in the funding gap for a variety of reasons. The United States, for example has its own AIDS relief program (PEPFAR—to be discussed below) that is more subject to U.S. political and religious values (concerning, for example, the use of generic drugs or condoms).

As a result, funding for AIDS projects is divided. Other problems that limit the effectiveness of GFATM often appear at the local level. Positive results include the training of health-care workers, the improvement of health-care clinics, and the provision of antiretroviral (ARV) drugs to people in need.[23]

WHO's 3X5 Program

On World AIDS Day 2003, the World Health Organization (WHO) and UNAIDS announced the details for implementing the ambitious "3X5 initiative"—providing antiretroviral treatment for three million people living with HIV/AIDS in developing countries by the end of the year 2005.

According to the plan, WHO will not buy the drugs but help governments by providing support and expertise. Partnerships with other global programs (for example, GFATM and PEPFAR) will help achieve the goals, including training one hundred thousand health workers, developing health-care systems, and building infrastructures to ensure a reliable supply of medicines.[24]

Although WHO announced that it met its 2004 goal of seven hundred thousand people, the 2005 goal of three million proved to be especially challenging. A major gap in funding led to a drastic reduction in its budget. It was reported that newly appointed staff "lured to WHO by the promise of resources to implement an ambitious treatment plan were shocked to learn that they would be expected to work miracles with no cash."[25]

By mid-2005 another report presented a nuanced view of the initiative:

> The 3 by 5 target is for half of all people in need of ARV drugs to be receiving them. This is not the same as each individual country reaching 50% coverage. Many of the worst affected nations had very low rates of provision when the initiative was launched, and access will remain unequal even if the December 2005 goal is achieved. Crucial to 3 by 5 success will be the progress of South Africa, India and Nigeria. At the end of

2004, these three nations between them accounted for 41% of unmet need. However, there are many countries which have severe HIV epidemics but whose achievements will have little effect on the total figures.[26]

Two other notes from this report: when India was a major producer of generic HIV/AIDS drugs, these drugs were affordable only by a tiny fraction of the people in India who needed treatment. In the United States, because of the lack of universal health care and because of cutbacks in federally and state-funded programs for AIDS, there are people who cannot get AIDS drugs—and so die.[27]

Clinton Foundation

The HIV/AIDS Initiative is a major component of the William J. Clinton Foundation. The initiative does not provide direct treatment, but it helps countries develop large-scale treatment and prevention programs by providing technical assistance and financial resources. It has succeeded in persuading drug-manufacturing companies to reduce the prices of the drugs, including generics, for sale to resource-limited countries. Some of the companies agreed to profit margins lower than normal.[28]

Numerous other foundations have become involved in promoting HIV/AIDS treatment and prevention programs, including the Bill and Melinda Gates Foundation, the Bristol-Myers Squibb Foundation, and the Henry J. Kaiser Family Foundation.

President's Emergency Plan for AIDS Relief

The President's Emergency Plan for AIDS Relief (PEPFAR) was announced in George Bush's 2003 State of the Union Address. It is a $15 billion, five-year plan to combat the HIV/AIDS epidemic outside the United States. (Other monies were requested for domestic programs.) The actual amount of money spent each year depends on what Congress appropriates for PEPFAR; in the first years it was less than $3 billion.

PEPFAR strongly emphasizes treatment and care for people with AIDS, with four-fifths of the money dedicated to this (including a significant percentage for the purchase and distribution of antiretroviral drugs) and only one-fifth for prevention. One-third of the prevention money must be spent on programs promoting sexual abstinence before marriage.

Another controversial aspect of PEPFAR is the limit placed on what products can be purchased. The plan requires that the drugs have FDA approval (or approval from a similar agency). This rules out some generics and Fixed Dose Combinations.

Despite these controversial aspects, along with the somewhat limited contribution to GFATM, PEPFAR has had a significant impact, especially in its focus countries, by supporting treatment programs with many millions of dollars.[29]

Despite the widespread influence and initial success of these programs and foundations, many people still hold onto misconceptions about costs and the AIDS epidemic. The authors of *Global AIDS: Myths and Facts* state what they consider one such misconception (myth) in this way:

> Financial resources for global health are extremely limited, so public health officials in poor countries should prioritize programs that address basic needs, such as nutrition, clean water, maternal health, and childhood immunization. Trying to provide costly, complicated AIDS treatment will divert an incredible share of countries' health budgets toward the needs of a few, while failing to deliver significant benefits for the rest of the populations.[30]

The authors acknowledge that many people in the world lack sufficient food and clean water and face serious health problems but argue that providing antiretroviral therapy will actually help poor countries' health programs. To substantiate their claim they discuss the following points: (1) HIV/AIDS demographics; (2) the consequences of AIDS on food production; (3) the relationship between AIDS and other infectious diseases; (4) the impact of the epidemic on children; and (5) AIDS and health care systems.[31]

(1) Because AIDS kills especially young adults, there are serious economic and social implications. Life expectancy is dropping sharply, threatening the affected countries' capacity for continued development and economic growth. ARV treatment can change this trend. "By stabilizing the workforce, slowing the loss of skills through illness and death, and helping secure the requirements for improved economic performance, AIDS treatment will benefit all of society and enable progress in other areas of health work." [32]

(2) The spread of HIV/AIDS is undermining agriculture in Africa. One problem follows another when a farm worker becomes ill: absence from work, absence of the caregiver from work, food must be purchased if no longer grown, and livestock suffers and may be sold off to cover expenses. In some countries in southern Africa agricultural production has been cut in half. Keeping farm workers strong is necessary for communities and countries. "Far from taking resources away from other, more fundamental health objectives, AIDS treatment in agricultural areas with high HIV/AIDS prevalence is necessary to ensure that people can meet the most basic health goal of all: getting enough food to eat."[33]

(3) Rather than taking a disproportionate share of poor countries' health budgets, AIDS treatment will help control other diseases, especially tuberculosis. Because of the strong connection between HIV and TB, ARV therapy will help control the spread of TB. AIDS treatment may also help reduce fear and stigma and promote good health attitudes.[34]

(4) The profound plight of children, especially orphans, has already been discussed in chapter 3. In the context of this threat to children's health and lives, it is clear that keeping the parents strong and productive (through ARV therapy) will greatly enhance the lives of many children. "The relatively high cost of anti-retroviral medications for parents with AIDS may be counterbalanced by significant benefits, not only for individual parents and children, who would be able to sustain their relationships over a longer time, but also for the community as a whole, whose stability would be enhanced by the reinforcement of family structures and the availability of greater material and social support for young people within families."[35]

(5) In high-prevalence countries, attempts to respond to AIDS-related diseases are overwhelming hospitals and clinics. Successful ARV-therapy programs will reduce this stress on health-care systems and allow attention to other illnesses.[36] The authors conclude, then, that a comprehensive health agenda can and must include ARV therapy. They recognize the financial costs, billions of dollars, but stress its cost-effectiveness when balanced against social and economic costs of not treating millions of people with HIV/AIDS. They contend that the resources exist. "The problem is not immovable structural constraints nor material scarcity, but how the affluent choose to spend money."[37]

The Consistent Ethic of Life responds well to this fundamental challenge concerning costs. As already described in chapter 2, church teachings emphasize that justice must be considered a constitutive dimension of the gospel. Individual and national acts of charity are necessary and good but not sufficient. Creating just policies and structures remains essential.

In their 1986 pastoral letter *Economic Justice for All* the U.S. bishops offer some foundational insights, rooted in the Scriptures and the social teachings, concerning ethics and economics—and so about this section's discussion of costs. As part of the pastoral letter, the bishops explain the contemporary phrase, "preferential option for the poor." The bishops point out that in the New Testament salvation is extended to all people. At the same time, Jesus takes the side of those most in need, physically and spiritually. The parable of the rich man and the poor Lazarus (Luke 16:19–31) is just one example of many in the Gospels that direct attention to the dangers of wealth. The rich are easily blinded by wealth and tempted to make it into an idol. While material poverty is certainly not good, the poor experience a dependence and powerlessness that may allow them more easily to be open to God's presence and power. Contemporary followers of Jesus, then, are challenged to take on this perspective: to see things from the side of the poor, to assess lifestyle and public policies in terms of their impact on the poor, and to experience God's power in the midst of poverty and powerlessness.[38]

Economic Justice for All highlights six basic moral principles to help guide economic choices and shape economic institutions: (1) every economic institution must be judged in light of whether it protects or undermines human dignity; (2) human dignity can be realized only in the community; (3) all people have a right to participate in the economic life of society; (4) all people have a special obligation to the poor; (5) human rights are the minimum conditions for life in community; and (6) society as a whole has the moral responsibility to enhance human dignity and protect human rights.[39]

Because of its wealth and power, the United States has a primary role in reforming the international economic order, particularly in relation to the developing world. It must work with other influential nations, with multilateral institutions, and with transnational banks and corporations. *Economic Justice for All* reviews five major areas where reform is needed and possible: (1) development assistance through grants, low-interest loans, and technical aid; (2) trade policy that is especially sensitive to the poorest nations; (3) international finance and investment,

with special attention to the Third World debt crisis; (4) private investment in foreign countries; and (5) an international food system that increases immediate food aid and develops long-term programs to combat hunger.[40]

The bishops acknowledge that their suggested reforms would be expensive. They also point to the immense human and social costs if reforms are not made. They judge that the amount of money spent on military purposes should be reduced, and some of this money should be
directed toward social and economic reforms. "In the end, the question
is not whether the United States can provide the necessary funds to meet
our social needs, but whether we have the political will to do so."[41] And
so they urge a new American experiment to complete the bold experiment in democracy begun more than two hundred years ago. This new
experiment in economic justice will demand a greater spirit of partnership and teamwork, a renewed commitment to the common good.[42]

Economic Justice for All, written during the first years of the AIDS
epidemic, still offers a penetrating analysis and challenging call to
wealthy nations, especially the United States. Will there be the political
will to turn away from war, armaments, and other instruments of the
culture of death and to turn toward partnership and the common good,
fully supporting programs like GFATM?

EDUCATIONAL PROGRAMS

*Is there a moral obligation concerning educational programs in light of
the growing epidemic?* Prevention remains the key to slowing the
spread of the HIV/AIDS pandemic. Most people recognize that education is a necessary dimension of promoting behavior change and prevention. The "ought" is clear, but not the "how."

In some cultures and countries, sexuality is still a taboo subject, particularly certain aspects of sexuality such as homosexuality. In some
cultures and countries, sexuality is everywhere, in entertainment and
advertising. In some cultures and countries, HIV/AIDS is largely de-
nied.

There are calls for educational prevention efforts to target preteens
before they become sexually active.[43] There are calls to help U.S. adolescents realize that sexual intimacy, "which carries rich significance

when sought within the bounds of permanent commitment to the full well-being of the beloved, is debased by a culture gone awry."[44]

How best to achieve these goals? In many cultures attention to oral means of communication rather than brochures and books is necessary. Dramas and workshops and especially peer education can be very effective.

This section, then, will focus on two aspects experienced in most situations and often discussed and debated: (1) education must be culturally sensitive and appropriate in order to be effective; and (2) education must include information about abstinence and condoms.

Education: Culturally Sensitive and Appropriate

Models of education based on wealthy nations' medical or religious views often fail to reach people at greatest risk of infection, whether in those wealthy countries or in the hardest-hit countries. A brief article by Tanzanian theologian and pastor Laurenti Magesa offers keen insight into this dilemma.[45]

Magesa begins by describing an encounter with one of his parishioners. Marcellus, in his forties, was dying of AIDS, as shown by his Kaposi's sarcoma. His first wife had already died. His relative's widow whom he "inherited" also showed symptoms of an AIDS-related disease. Magesa notes: "This was all circumstantial evidence, of course, but in many rural areas of Africa, and certainly in Bukama, it is often all we have to go by in the way of prognosis."[46]

Marcellus was convinced that his illness was due to a "bad wind" caused by people who wished him evil. He was convinced that no Western medicine could help, though an African type probably could. Marcellus gave directions to Magesa about his burial, and a week later Marcellus died.

Magesa begins his analysis boldly: Marcellus "illustrates a situation prevalent across sub-Saharan Africa where injunctions to abstain from sexual relations, or to be faithful in monogamous unions, or even to use condoms as protective and preventive measures against HIV/AIDS transmission, will not much succeed in the African person's cultural context."[47]

Why? Magesa offers two reasons: African people interpret HIV/AIDS in terms of their cultural world as a breach of a taboo and witchcraft, and they understand sexuality and sexual activity to be geared toward marriage and procreation, preserving the clan's life force.

As was evident in Marcellus's case, the common belief is that HIV/AIDS is caused by some evil spirit or witch. Magesa points out that such belief is also found among the educated and even medically trained: priests, nuns, and nurses. "Accusations of witchcraft and suspicions about casting the 'evil eye' still occasionally surface in the parishes and convents."[48]

Because of their conviction that procreation preserves the life force (and so immortality), many African people practice polygamy, widow inheritance, and widow-cleansing (a widow is required to have sexual relations with one of her deceased husband's relatives)—all high-risk practices. Magesa states that sexuality and birth are about the bonding of the visible and invisible worlds, about protecting the widow, and about assuring the continuation of the life of the clan.

> To disturb this purpose in any way means to tamper dangerously with human life, God, the spirits, and the ancestors. If the lineage is to die because a person refuses to fulfill his or her responsibility in this regard, the person in question commits a grave offense against God and the ancestors. Such behavior can bring about untold calamities, not only for the individual concerned, but often also for the entire community. For this reason, the requirement to observe these sexual customs is in many cases weightier in the eyes of the people than the risk of acquiring HIV/AIDS which arises from these customs.[49]

In this context, what kind of education is necessary? Magesa claims that neither "the biomedical paradigm which says 'Treat your Sexually Transmitted Diseases (STDs), use condoms and change your sexual behavior in order to survive'" nor "the Christian-missionary approach which preaches against the use of condoms and insists on abstinence"[50] will be effective. Only an approach that starts within traditional ideas and the perceived tradition will be heard and accepted.

For Magesa and his African context, this approach would begin with the beliefs in witchcraft as the cause of illness and in sexuality as a means to enhance life and use their ethical demands to promote behavior change. The first step is to help others recognize the witchcraft within themselves, that is, the propensity to wrongdoing. Controlling this propensity in a time of AIDS means not risking harm to yourself by avoiding promiscuity.

Magesa suggests a similar insight regarding sexuality.

If the use of sexuality in African culture is oriented toward solidarity of
the community, that is, by enhancing the life force of the living, the dead,
and the yet to be born through procreation, anything or any behavior that
obstructs this contradicts the sense of life and cannot be encouraged by
the community. When African communities, therefore, are made to realize that some of their marriage institutions and sexual rituals do in fact di-
minish rather than promote the life of the community, because they are
agents of death, they may more easily be persuaded to transcend and
change them.[51]

The heart of Magesa's insights can be applied in many different situations around the world, demanding of course a deep appreciation of the
local cultural and religious worldviews. Culturally responsive education
could then be developed for men who have sex with men in cultures that
deny homosexuality, for women who have little or no freedom in matters of sexuality, and for groups of those addicted to drugs or at risk of
addiction. "Any effective change begins with addressing people's
worldview."[52]

Education: Abstinence and Condoms

Magesa's article has already named two different models (the biomedical paradigm and the Christian-missionary approach) that have sparked
much debate. Does education for prevention focus on condoms or abstinence?

In fact, the fundamental approach to education for prevention includes both and has been called simply the ABC method popularized in
Uganda: **A**bstain, **B**e faithful, Use **C**ondoms. Nevertheless, debate
about emphasizing one more than the other has continued throughout
the years of the epidemic's spread, with some groups focusing on condom distribution and other groups promoting abstinence. Often the debate reflects a deeper difference in worldviews or ideologies, coloring
both articles and reports.

Three events can serve as examples of this long debate. As briefly described in chapter 3, a conflict developed among the Catholic bishops
in the United States after the publication of *The Many Faces of AIDS* because this statement suggested a context in which information about

condoms could be given. Some bishops were concerned that this comment about condoms would compromise Catholic teaching and so confuse the faithful. This internal debate led to the bishops' conference publishing a second statement, *Called to Compassion and Responsibility*, which stressed official Church teaching on sexuality and said that the use of condoms to prevent the spread of HIV is technically unreliable and morally unacceptable.[53]

The second event was President Bush's funding of PEPFAR. As was indicated earlier in this chapter, one-third of the money for prevention must be spent on programs promoting abstinence before marriage. Some people objected to this focus on abstinence; others complained that two-thirds of the money did not necessarily focus on abstinence!

The third event was a meeting at the Fifteenth International AIDS Conference in Bangkok. The meeting was billed as "CNN vs. ABC"— Condoms, Needles, and Negotiation skills vs. Abstain, Be faithful, or Use Condoms. Opposing sides emphasized different points, even while acknowledging some agreement. "CNN" claimed that condom promotion is clearly effective in some situations (but needs lots of effort to educate people in effective use) and that abstinence-only education lacked clear evidence that it works. "ABC" claimed that there was no evidence in Africa that more condoms meant less AIDS and that the reduction in Uganda occurred because of delayed sex among young people and fewer extramarital relationships.[54]

So the debate continues!

The biomedical model takes a pragmatic approach, recognizing that people will continue to engage in many forms of sexual activity. Condoms can reduce the risk of HIV transmission, though not eliminate it. The long debate has also included exchanges about the effectiveness of condoms.[55]

The religiously-based model sees the use of condoms as contradicting the meaning of sexuality and perhaps as intrinsically evil. Condoms become a "technofix"[56] and fail to address underlying behavioral and cultural issues.

> How much have we accomplished if we teach a wife to use a condom to prevent her becoming infected by her husband, who is continuing to engage in sexual intercourse with commercial sex workers, if we pay no attention to the culturally based support for such behavior on his part? Analogously, while we clearly want to protect the lives of women who for

whatever reasons are engaged in prostitution, we must also examine the double standards which exist for men and women in societies around the world which place wives at risk and which lead to the trafficking of women and children as sex objects.[57]

These wider concerns move the discussion from either condoms or abstinence to a more inclusive ABC model in a context of cultural, economic, and political awareness (these latter issues will be discussed in the next chapter).

In his essay reflecting on Uganda's experience, Dr. Edward C. Green, a member of the U.S. Presidential Advisory Council on HIV and AIDS, stressed the complete ABC approach and not abstinence only. However, his reading of the data emphasized that the declining rates of HIV infection in Uganda were due primarily to A and B. Studies show that people listened to their president's simple, direct message: "Stop having multiple partners. Be faithful. Teenagers, wait until you are married before you begin sex."[58] Widespread availability of condoms happened after the decline had started.

Green acknowledges that his perspective is met with suspicion but claims that studies reveal that Africans speak about becoming monogamous when describing their change of behavior in response to HIV/AIDS.

> The ABC approach is not about that great conversation-stopper, 'abstinence only.' It is about providing people with more options for preventing AIDS. Some people cannot or will not change their behavior, and so of course they need to use condoms. But while condom use was one of the options Uganda has promoted, faithfulness to one partner is probably the major contributor to the country's success. We need to develop a balanced approach by recognizing that Africa and the West have different types of epidemics and going beyond the fruitless battle between the abstinence and condom camps.[59]

Using the Ugandan data along with other studies, a group of AIDS researchers has concluded that the B of ABC has been seriously neglected. Still, "Be faithful," especially when understood broadly to include reductions in casual sex and the number of partners, has been very effective in reducing the rate of HIV infection. The authors point out that a significant aspect of this behavior change is that it was accompanied by changes in group norms of behavior.

In Uganda, a combination of explicit and repeated presidential pronouncements and the committed engagement of faith based organizations, the governmental apparatus, the military, the health system, and community based and mass communications—all in the context of the stark reality of people dying from AIDS—seem to have achieved a "tipping point" so that avoiding risky sex has become the community norm. This experience supports the need for reinforcing messages from multiple sources. In addition, most of the behaviour change approaches originated within Uganda (and similarly within Thailand), suggesting external assistance should reinforce such locally developed approaches.[60]

A consensus statement signed in 2004 by more than 140 AIDS experts expressed strong and nuanced support for ABC and called for an end to the polarizing debate. While acknowledging the growing problem of injecting drug use, the statement focused on preventing sexually transmitted HIV.

It recommended three key principles. First, programs for education and prevention must be culturally and socially sensitive, based on epidemiological evidence and respectful of human rights.

Second, the ABC approach can play a significant part in slowing the spread of HIV.

All three elements of this approach are essential to reducing HIV incidence, although the emphasis placed on individual elements needs to vary according to the target population. Although the overall programmatic mix should include an appropriate balance of A, B, and C interventions, it is not essential that every organization promote all three elements: each can focus on the part(s) they are most comfortable supporting. However, all people should have accurate and complete information about different prevention options, including all three elements of the ABC approach.[61]

Third, community-based approaches involving local organizations can develop new norms for sexual behavior (as happened in Uganda). In this context, prevention programs "need to address issues such as stigma, gender inequality, sexual coercion, cross-generational relationships and transactional sex, and directly involve people living with HIV/AIDS" in order to achieve the goals for behavioral change.[62]

The statement ends by urging greatly expanded availability of testing, counseling, and treating and by recommending attention to new methods of prevention.

Former U.S. Surgeon General David Satcher has added an important note to the ABC model—a component of hope. Satcher stated that "any domestic version of an ABC approach must be expanded to also address the sense of hopelessness that too often leads many people to engage in high-risk sexual behavior."[63]

As discussed in chapter 3, the differing Catholic perspectives on the use of condoms to prevent the spread of HIV are rooted in different moral methodologies and different worldviews, often described as "classicist" or "modern/historical," that also lead to differing understandings of the relationship between conscience and authority.[64] For now the differences remain. Magesa's concluding words seem to fit here as well: "Any effective change begins with addressing people's worldviews."[65]

SUPPORT FOR PROGRAMS

Should programs that promote the use of condoms or needle exchange be supported? While the previous question focused more on educational programs aimed at prevention of the transmission of HIV, the heated debate spills over into the discussion about practical programs of prevention. Should condoms and clean needles be distributed as a way of combating HIV/AIDS? Because some religious groups and other organizations see condom distribution and use as promoting irresponsible and immoral sexual activity, they have opposed the C in ABC. Others see condoms as a proven means of reducing the transmission of HIV. All of this was clearly indicated in the previous question.

So, for this question, focus can be given to the issue of needle exchange (providing sterile needles and syringes in place of contaminated ones; an already used needle or syringe may have infected blood in it). The religious groups just mentioned often evaluate needle-exchange programs in a similar way: they promote an illegal and immoral practice and so must not be supported.[66]

The U.S. federal government also opposes needle exchange programs. Again, the reason given is that such programs would be promoting illegal behavior and send the wrong message about drug abuse. Most states, however, do support needle-exchange programs but cannot use federal funds for these programs.

Many people in the scientific community point to the growing evidence (more than two hundred studies) that such programs in fact reduce the spread of HIV and do not promote drug use.[67] Many programs offer not only clean needles but also drug treatment referrals, methadone clinics, peer education, and HIV prevention programs. In doing so, they fit the "harm reduction criteria" developed by WHO and UNAIDS.[68]

Why the urgency of this debate? Because injecting drug use is the cause of over 50 percent of AIDS cases in some countries, an estimated 70 percent in Russia. It is also a serious problem in U.S. cities. The use of illegal drugs is often connected with other social problems, especially poverty and marginalization. An "escape" leads to addiction and a whole host of illegal and dangerous activities. Users often share their equipment, resulting in the possibility of injecting with the drugs some infected blood, a highly efficient means of HIV transmission. Infected drug users may then infect their sexual partners and often their children. Thus the epidemic spreads.

Why the resistance? Once again it seems to be a conflict of worldviews, despite evidence that the programs are effective in lessening HIV transmission and cost-effective too, despite attempts to demonstrate that the Catholic tradition can support needle exchange.

Jorge J. Ferrer, S.J., for example, carefully analyzes needle-exchange programs from the perspective of two traditional principles, cooperation and counseling the lesser of two evils. Using these principles he concludes that needle exchange not only is justified but maybe even obligatory.[69] Other theologians use other approaches to reach similar conclusions. Nevertheless, these arguments fail to convince, and opposition continues.[70]

EFFECTS OF PREJUDICE

What about the effects of prejudice against HIV-infected persons and their families and friends in housing, parishes, employment, insurance, and medical treatment? Stigmatization has been and remains a major issue in the HIV/AIDS pandemic. In a great variety of cultures, countries, and religions, HIV-positive people find their human rights limited and violated. Some literally lose their lives to violence rooted in fear and prejudice. Many others fail to seek out testing and treatment because of fear of experiencing stigmatization. Such prejudice flourishes despite the fact that many organizations and countries have emphasized human rights since the beginning of the epidemic.[71]

Several examples can only hint at the stigmatization experienced by so many people.

In his book *HIV, AIDS & Islam*, Farid Esack tells the story of Nabil, an Arab Muslim who injected drugs and had sex with other men. He did not think that HIV/AIDS could affect him personally. But a medical test that was required before he began a new job in Miami revealed that he was HIV-positive. The company refused to hire him. His family living in Amman, Jordan, rejected him. His father would not allow his sisters to speak Nabil's name; the sisters told Nabil to read the Qur'an.

Eventually, Nabil did find help through a New York City organization called MENTORS (Middle East Natives Testing, Orientation and Referral Service). "Some fellow Arabs and Muslims treated me well and accepted me the way I am," said Nabil. "They accepted my humanity, and this reversed my view of life, and my role in it."[72] As a result, before he died, Nabil worked to educate other Arabs and Muslims about HIV/AIDS and to combat the widespread perception that the disease did not affect them.[73]

A very different example is described by Ann Smith and Enda Mc-Donagh. The HIV-related discrimination faced by Rwandan refugees seeking a new life in the USA after the genocide provides a stark example of the denial of human rights and human dignity.

In the late 1990s the United States agreed to welcome a number of refugees from Rwanda. Part of the preparation for their application process was a medical examination including an HIV test. Those found to be positive were excluded. If the person excluded had other family members also applying, all were refused on the basis that families need to stay together. Yet one can assume that the original asylum offer from USA (and other countries have similar policies) was made to these people because of their vulnerability and the trauma which they experienced in the genocide of 1994.

The trauma of many Rwandan women was intensified by their discovery that, when they were raped, they had also been infected with HIV. To some extent those living with the virus could be seen as being more vulnerable than those not infected and most in need of humanitarian assistance, and yet these are the very people refused.74

A famous early example of discrimination was the case of Ryan White. He was a teenager from Kokomo, Indiana, who had hemophilia. In the early 1980s, some blood products made for hemophiliacs contained HIV, so many became infected.

Some excerpts from White's own testimony before the President's Commission on AIDS give some sense of his experience. "I came face to face with death at thirteen years old. . . . It was my decision to live a normal life, go to school, be with friends. . . . The school board, my teachers, and my principal voted to keep me out of the classroom . . . for fear of someone getting AIDS from me by casual contact. Rumors of sneezing, kissing, tears, sweat, and saliva spreading AIDS caused people to panic."75

White goes on to describe the legal battle to attend school and the concessions he and his mother made with the school: "separate restrooms, no gym, separate drinking fountains, disposable eating utensils and trays."

"Nevertheless, parents of twenty students started their own school. . . . Because of the lack of education on AIDS, discrimination, fear, panic, and lies surrounded me. . . . People would get up and leave so they would not have to sit anywhere near me. Even at church, people would not shake my hand."76

Media focused on his case, and soon Ryan White became a celebrity. Eventually, he was accepted by a new school, Hamilton Heights High School, in Cicero, Indiana. Ryan White died in 1990 at the age of 18.

Ryan White, of course, is a most unusual example in that most people do not have films made about them nor do they have federal legislation named after them. Some commentators contend that White got so much attention because as a white, middle-class, heterosexual boy he was not part of the minority groups stigmatized by HIV/AIDS. Indeed, the use of "innocent victims" continues for certain groups of HIV-positive people, revealing an ongoing prejudice.

The final example comes from a UNAIDS report in 2005 on AIDS in Asia and the Pacific.77 This report states: "Perhaps the greatest obstacle to a successful response is that stigma and discrimination against people living with HIV remain the norm in many Asian countries. For instance, high levels of HIV-related stigma and discrimination deter many individuals from accessing the services they need."78

The report goes on to say that a significant percentage of HIV-positive people have experienced discrimination in health-care settings, including breakdowns in confidentiality and even refusal of treatment.

Although numerous countries in the area have expressed commitment to protect human rights, in practice specific legal measures and structures are lacking.[79]

Despite the official emphasis on human rights, stigmatization continues to spread with the pandemic around the globe. There is, then, a clear need for education and behavioral change, leading people and societies to recognize and overcome prejudice.

Efforts to overcome prejudice of course are notoriously difficult to implement successfully. Laws are essential, but so much more is necessary. Understanding, openness, and contact with "the other" are especially helpful in breaking down barriers. The role of government, then, is necessary but not sufficient. Nongovernmental agencies are often more successful in making connections between people. Religions can have a profound influence, either in reinforcing the prejudice or in overcoming it.

Some religious leaders have described HIV/AIDS as God's punishment for sin (for example, homosexuality). Others, following Jesus's example as described in chapter 2, have stressed compassion, human rights, and the need to change oppressive structures of society.

Although there remains debate in the Catholic community about condoms and needle-exchange programs, statements from the Vatican and from bishops' groups have consistently denounced discrimination and prejudice. An excerpt from one of John Paul II's many speeches on HIV/AIDS strongly expresses this conviction.

AIDS threatens not just some nations or societies but the whole of humanity. It knows no frontiers of geography, race, age or social condition. . . . The threat is so great that indifference on the part of public authorities, condemnatory or discriminatory practices towards those affected by the virus or self-interested rivalries in the search for a medical answer to this syndrome should be considered forms of collaboration in this terrible evil which has come upon humanity.[80]

A similar position is clearly stated in the two documents from the U.S. bishops. *The Many Faces of AIDS* says directly: "Discrimination or violence directed against persons with AIDS is unjust and immoral"[81] and also "All human life is sacred, and its dignity must be respected and protected."[82]

The statement goes on to apply these comments to specific situations. It opposes quarantine and widespread mandatory testing. It urges legislators to act judiciously and not out of hysteria or prejudice. While recognizing the complexity of insurance issues, it condemns the exclusion of HIV-positive persons from health insurance and uses the occasion to promote accessible health care for all. It calls upon health-care professionals to provide care in their field for infected persons. It encourages protection against discrimination in housing, education, and employment.[83]

Called to Compassion and Responsibility reaffirmed all these key points. Without explicitly using the language of the Consistent Ethic of Life, these and other statements have expressed its essential principles and insights concerning the continuing problem of stigmatization.

These complex societal responsibilities often point to the even more complex and challenging global structural issues to which we now turn.

NOTES

1. Robert J. Blendon, Karen Donelan, and Richard A. Knox, "Public Opinion and AIDS," in *AIDS, Ethics & Religion*, ed. Kenneth R. Overberg, S.J. (Maryknoll, N.Y.: Orbis Books, 1994), 143–57.

2. For a variety of perspectives, see James F. Keenan, S.J., ed., *Catholic Ethicists on HIV/AIDS Prevention* (New York: Continuum, 2000), 41–107, especially Laurenti Magesa, "Recognizing the Reality of African Religion in Tanzania," 76–84.

3. Tom Fawthrop, "Cuba: Is It a Model in HIV-AIDS Battle?" *Global Policy Forum*, www.globalpolicy.org/socecon/develop/aids/2003/12cuba.htm (accessed 21 November 2005).

4. Ronald Bayer, "Public Health Policy and the AIDS Epidemic: An End to HIV Exceptionalism?" in *AIDS, Ethics*, ed. Overberg, 170–71.

5. Bayer, "Public Health," 174.

6. Marcia Angell, "A Dual Approach to the AIDS Epidemic," in *AIDS, Ethics*, ed. Overberg, 178–82.

7. Angell, "Dual Approach," 181.

8. David E. Rogers and June E. Osborn, "Another Approach to the AIDS Epidemic," in *AIDS, Ethics*, ed. Overberg, 183–88.

9. Rogers and Osborn, "Another Approach," 184.

10. Rogers and Osborn, "Another Approach," 185–87.

11. National Conference of Catholic Bishops, *Called to Compassion and Responsibility* (Washington, D.C.: USCC Office of Publishing Services, 1990), 24–25.

12. National Conference, *Called to Compassion*, 21–22.

13. National Conference, *Called to Compassion*, 24.

14. National Conference, *Called to Compassion*, 25.

15. Jane Pennington, "Voluntary, Routine and Mandatory HIV Testing," *AVERT*, www.avert.org/hiv~test.htm (accessed 20 June 2005).

16. *El Comercio*, "HIV/AIDS Tests?" *Human Rights Watch*, hrw.org/english/docs/2004/05/14peru8584txt.htm (accessed 20 June 2005).

17. *El Comercio*, "HIV/AIDS Tests?"

18. Tripti Tandon, "Mandatory Testing, HIV/AIDS and Marriage—Discordant Bedfellows?" *Lawyers Collective*, www.lawyerscollective.org/lc-hiv-aids/magazine_articles/may_2002.htm (accessed 20 June 2005).

19. UNAIDS, "Bringing Comprehensive HIV Prevention to Scale," *2004 Report on the Global AIDS Epidemic,* www.unaids.org/bangkok2004 (accessed 21 June 2005).

20. AIDS Action Council, "Policy Facts: Incarcerated Populations and HIV/AIDS," *The Body*, www.thebody.com/aac/brochures/incarcerated.html (accessed 21 June 2005).

21. Ralf Jurgens, "HIV Testing and Confidentiality: Final Report," *Canadian HIV/AIDS Legal Network,* www.aidslaw.ca/Maincontent/issues/testing/07mandate1.html (accessed 21 June 2005).

22. Office of the High Commissioner for Human Rights and UNAIDS, "HIV/AIDS and Human Rights: International Guidelines," *UNAIDS*, www.unaids.org/en/default.asp, then use search for "HIV/AIDS and Human Rights: International Guidelines" (accessed 22 June 2005).

23. Bonita deBoer, "The Global Fund to Fight AIDS, Tuberculosis and Malaria," *AVERT*, www.avert.org/global-fund.htm (accessed 23 June 2005).

24. World Health Organization, "The 3 by 5 Initiative," *WHO*, www.who.int/3by5/about/en (accessed 23 June 2005).

25. Keith Alcorn, "UNAIDS Envoy Raises Alarm over Funding for 3X5," *NAM*, www.aidsmap.com/en/news163A590D6-4357-4D2C-9038-3D2BA564E456.asp (accessed 23 June 2005).

26. Avert, "AIDS Treatment: Targets and Results," *AVERT*, www.avert.org/aidstarget.htm (accessed 23 June 2005).

27. Avert, "AIDS Treatment."

28. Clinton Foundation, "HIV/AIDS Initiative," *Clinton Foundation*, www.clintonfoundation.org/cf-pgm-hs-ai-home.htm (accessed 23 June 2005).

29. Annabel Kanabus, "President's Emergency Plan for AIDS Relief," *AVERT*, www.avert.org/pepfar.htm (accessed 23 June 2005).

30. Alexander Irwin, Joyce Millen, and Dorothy Fallows, *Global AIDS: Myths and Facts* (Cambridge, Mass.: South End Press, 2003), 135.

31. Irwin, Millen, and Fallows, *Global AIDS*, 136–48.

32. Irwin, Millen, and Fallows, *Global AIDS*, 138.

33. Irwin, Millen, and Fallows, *Global AIDS*, 140.

34. Irwin, Millen, and Fallows, *Global AIDS*, 141–42.

35. Irwin, Millen, and Fallows, *Global AIDS*, 145–46.

36. Irwin, Millen, and Fallows, *Global AIDS*, 146–48.

37. Irwin, Millen, and Fallows, *Global AIDS*, 150.

38. National Conference of Catholic Bishops, *Economic Justice for All* (Washington, D.C.: USCC Office of Publishing Services, 1986), 26–29 (para. 48–52).

39. NCCB, *Economic Justice*, 6–11 (para. 12–22).

40. NCCB, *Economic Justice*, 126–40 (or para. 261–87).

41. NCCB, *Economic Justice*, 143 (or para. 294).

42. NCCB, *Economic Justice*, 145–47 (or para. 295–97).

43. H. Vandenhoudt, "First Sexual Intercourse and Exposure to HIV Infection among Young Women in a High Prevalence Area in Western Kenya" (paper presented at the XV International AIDS Conference, Bangkok, July 2004).

44. Stephen G. Post, "Adolescents in a Time of AIDS," *America*, vol. 167, no. 11 (October 17, 1992): 279.

45. Laurenti Magesa, "Recognizing the Reality of African Religion in Tanzania," in *Catholic Ethicists on HIV/AIDS Prevention*, ed. James F. Keenan, S.J. (New York: Continuum, 2000), 76–84.

46. Magesa, "Recognizing," 77.

47. Magesa, "Recognizing," 77–78.

48. Magesa, "Recognizing," 79.

49. Magesa, "Recognizing," 80.

50. Magesa, "Recognizing," 80–81.

51. Magesa, "Recognizing," 83.

52. Magesa, "Recognizing," 84.

53. NCCB, *Called to Compassion*, 20; for more, see the Introduction in *Catholic Ethicists on HIV/AIDS Prevention*, 21–25.

54. Julian Meldrum, "Abstinence Debate Finds More Consensus than Difference," *NAM*, www.aidsmap.com/en/news/FD76F652-0004-4E67-BF0C-E69BD4E94440.asp (accessed 27 June 2005).

55. Keenan, S.J., *Catholic Ethicists*, 24–25.

56. Post, "Adolescents," 278.

57. Keenan, S.J., *Catholic Ethicists*, 35.

58. Edward C. Green, "The New AIDS Fight: A Plan as Simple as ABC," *New York Times*, 1 March 2003.

59. Green, "New AIDS Fight."

60. James Shelton, Daniel Halperin, Vinand Nantulya, Malcolm Potts, Helene Gayle, and King Holmes, "Partner Reduction Is Crucial for Balanced 'ABC' Approach to HIV Prevention," *British Medical Journal*, no. 328 (10 April 2004): 892.

61. Daniel T. Halperin, et al., "The Time Has Come for Common Ground on Preventing Sexual Transmission of HIV," *The Lancet*, no. 364 (27 Nov 2004): 1914.

62. Halperin, "Time Has Come," 1914.

63. David Satcher, "ABC & Hope Approach to HIV Prevention" (paper presented at the conference "The Call to Action on Sexual Health," Morehouse School of Medicine, May 2004).

64. Richard M. Gula, S.S., *Reason Informed by Faith* (Mahwah, N.J.: Paulist Press, 1989), 30–36 and 123–62. Also see Kenneth R. Overberg, S.J., *Conscience in Conflict,* third edition (Cincinnati: St. Anthony Messenger Press, 2006), especially chapter 3.

65. Magesa, "Recognizing," 84.

66. For example: NCCB, *Called to Compassion*, 18–20.

67. World Health Organization, "Policy Brief: Provision of Sterile Injecting Equipment to Reduce HIV Transmission," *WHO*, www.wpro.who.int/NR/rdonlyres/BA463DB4-2390-4964-9D86-11CBABCC9DA9/0/provisionofsterlieen.pdf (accessed 28 June 2005).

68. UNAIDS, "The Warsaw Declaration: A Framework for Effective Action on HIV/AIDS and Injecting Drug Use," *UNAIDS*, www.unaids.org/en/default.asp, then use search for "The Warsaw Declaration" (accessed 28 June 2005).

69. Jorge J. Ferrer, S.J., "Needle Exchange in San Juan, Puerto Rico: A Traditional Roman Catholic Casuistic Approach," in Keenan, S.J., *Catholic Ethicists*, 177–91.

70. See Keenan, S.J., *Catholic Ethicists*, 26–29 and 35–36.

71. Jonathan Mann, Daniel J. M. Tarantola, and Thomas W. Netter, eds., *AIDS in the World* (Cambridge, Mass.: Harvard University Press, 1992), 561–73.

72. Farid Esack, *HIV, AIDS & Islam* (Observatory, South Africa: Positive Muslims, 2004), 14.

73. Esack, *AIDS & Islam*, 14–15.

74. Ann Smith and Enda McDonagh, *The Reality of HIV/AIDS* (Maynooth, Ireland: Trocaire, Veritas, CAFOD, 2003), 75.

75. Ryan White, "Testimony before the President's Commission on AIDS," *Wikisource*, en.wikisource.org/wiki/Ryan_White's_Testimony_before_the_President's_Commission_on_AIDS (accessed 1 July 2005), 1.

76. White, "Testimony," 2.

77. UNAIDS, "A Scaled Up Response to AIDS in Asia and the Pacific" (report given at the 7th International Congress on AIDS in Asia and the Pacific, Kobe, Japan, 1–5 July 2005).

78. UNAIDS, "AIDS in Asia and the Pacific," 27.

79. UNAIDS, "AIDS in Asia and the Pacific," 27.

80. Pope John Paul II, "The AIDS Epidemic," *Origins*, vol. 20, no. 15 (20 September 1990): 242–43.

81. Administrative Board of the United States Catholic Conference, *The Many Faces of AIDS* (Washington, D.C.: USCC Office of Publishing Services, 1987), 2.

82. USCC, *Many Faces*, 5.

83. USCC, *Many Faces*, 9–12.

Chapter Seven

Ethics and Global Structures

HIV and AIDS raise ethical questions that extend throughout the life cycle and around the globe. In this chapter, we will consider the fifth cluster of these questions concerning the global structural issues. More accurately, it is one basic question about a cluster of issues: *What ought governments and other organizations do about the economic and social and political structures that contribute to behavior that could spread HIV?* Poverty, racism, oppression of women, globalization and the maximization of profits, forced migration, and war and violence of all kinds create the perfect breeding grounds (risky sexual situations and the injection of drugs) for the growth of the HIV/AIDS epidemic. What ought governments and other organizations do to respond, and how can individual persons help?

Most if not all of the questions we have already considered are influenced and even created by these structural issues. To confront the AIDS pandemic adequately, then, demands addressing these often overwhelming problems that John Paul II called "structures of sin."[1] This chapter will first consider in some detail these social and economic structures and then develop a response rooted in the Consistent Ethic of Life.

POVERTY

"Ours is a highly unequal and unjust world and nowhere is this more evident than in relation to HIV/AIDS. In rich countries, advances made in antiretroviral drugs and other means of ensuring care and well-being have meant that many of those living with HIV/AIDS continue to live active and productive lives. . . In some developing countries, meanwhile, life expectancies are back to rates last seen in Europe in medieval times."[2]

Ann Smith and Enda McDonagh go on to describe succinctly the vicious cycle of poverty and AIDS. "While poverty does not cause HIV/AIDS, it facilitates transmission, makes adequate treatment impossible to afford, accelerates death from AIDS-related illness and multiplies the social impact of the epidemic."[3] Poverty makes a person much more vulnerable, generally because of poorer health, fewer health services, less awareness of HIV education, and greater possibility of risky sexual encounters that provide means to help meet immediate needs (such as food, shelter, or school fees).

At the same time, especially in the developing world, HIV makes poverty even worse. For individual families, it reduces income as wage earners get sick and die. Children drop out of school. Resources are used up for medicines and funerals. For societies, employment and development decline. As we saw in the previous chapter, the deaths of so many young adults undermine teaching, agriculture, health-care systems, and the care of both elders and children.[4]

Let one story symbolize millions.[5] Nsanga, a woman in her twenties with two children, had been married to a schoolteacher. Because of structural adjustment measures instituted by the International Monetary Fund (IMF), the government of Zaire (now the Democratic Republic of Congo) was forced to make cutbacks in its expenses, including laying off teachers and health workers. Nsanga's husband lost his job, was not able to find a new one, began spending their small resources on drinking, and finally simply disappeared.

Nsanga was very poor, as were her living conditions.

[She lived in a] single room which was part of a corrugated-roofed block surrounding an open courtyard. The yard contained a shared water tap, a roofless bathing stall, and a latrine, but no electricity. In good weather Nsanga and her neighbors moved their charcoal stoves outdoors to cook. In the courtyard, they also washed dishes and clothes and prepared vegetables for the pot. Wastewater ran out to an open ditch outside. Like the yard, the street was unpaved, deeply rutted, muddy in the rainy season, and dusty in the dry months. Mosquitoes were ubiquitous in the neighborhood, and malaria and diarrheal diseases were common causes of death in young children. Many families ate only one meal per day and children were especially undernourished. Many people had deep, hacking coughs that suggested pulmonary tuberculosis.[6]

Nsanga, like most poor women in Kinshasa (the capital city with a population of several million people), had only a few years of education in primary school. She unsuccessfully tried to find employment and so did small jobs in the neighborhood. These were not enough to pay for rent and food, so Nsanga began exchanging sex for subsistence. For a year, her lover was a married man who paid her rent. After she became pregnant, he left her, so Nsanga had to find more partners. At the time, the "neighborhood rate was equivalent to U.S. fifty cents per brief encounter,"[7] so two partners per day would produce about $30 a month.

Nsanga's medical history included an earlier ectopic pregnancy that led to a blood transfusion. She had symptoms of a sexually transmitted disease but had no money to consult a doctor. Condoms were for "prostitutes," and she was not one of those but only a mother trying to fulfill her obligations.

"Abandonment, divorce, and widowhood force many women who are without other resources into commercial sex work. In the presence of HIV, however, this survival strategy has been transformed into a death strategy."[8]

Nsanga's story points to the pervasive power of poverty. It also highlights the impact of socioeconomic and political conditions, including the consequences of IMF policies and the cultural oppression of women. It reveals how difficult it is to change what people consider normal behavior, leading the author to call for "culturally appropriate, interactive, community-based change strategies"[9] and not just targeted information campaigns or education. Schoepf concludes:

> AIDS prevention involves much more than the adoption of condoms or reduction in partner numbers. Rather, it involves redefinition of the gendered social roles and change in the socioeconomic conditions that have contributed to the rapid spread of HIV in Africa. Its rapid spread through heterosexual transmission in other regions of the world confirms this hypothesis. Success in the quest for AIDS prevention mandates the use of social empowerment strategies and demands changes in development goals to put people—rather than production, profit, and professional advance—first.[10]

RACISM

HIV/AIDS' preferential option for the poor expresses itself in the United States with high rates of infection among people of color. Many of these communities already experience prejudice, poverty, crime, and injecting drug abuse. As we already saw in chapter 4, "HIV is sweeping through black communities in the South, where stigma, inadequate medical care and poverty hamper efforts to educate and prevent its spread."[11]

In the South and throughout the country, racism and its long history continue to harm people. African-American and Hispanic women, for example, represent less than one-quarter of all women in the United States but account for about 80 percent of AIDS cases among women. Public health professionals claim that minorities are less likely to experience HIV education programs, to be tested, and to have access to health care.

For a conference on AIDS and religion in America sponsored by the Council of Religious AIDS Networks, Reverend Joseph R. Barndt addressed the interrelationship of racism and AIDS.[12] Barndt, former executive director of Crossroads, an interfaith ministry in Chicago for racial justice, claims that for adequate understanding of the intimate relationship between racism and AIDS it is first necessary to begin with basic presuppositions about racism.

Barndt suggests three: (1) "Racism is a systemic issue, more than personal and relational."[13] He says that people of color are hurt more by white institutions than by white individuals. (2) "The end goal of racism is white power and privilege."[14] Harm done to people of color is the consequence of racism but not its purpose. Racism's goal is helping and empowering white society. (3) "Racism is preserved in the roots of every U.S. institution. Racism is like a weed that thrives in its roots even after the visible plant is torn from the ground."[15] Therefore, it is necessary to deal with discrimination's underlying causes.

Relating these presuppositions to the HIV/AIDS epidemic, Barndt moves beyond individual expressions of prejudice to focus on racism in the health-care system and how this system has acted in preferential ways for white people. "The problem is not simply the interrelationship of racism and AIDS, but that People of Color are now and have always been disproportionately without access to, resources from, and control over every aspect related to a just and affordable health care system."[16]

He recommends a two-pronged response: to confront discriminatory practices and policies at every opportunity and to adopt an antiracist understanding toward the entire health-care system. "Fundamental change in the cure and treatment of HIV/AIDS is interdependent with—and cannot be separated from—the struggle to transform the racism of the entire health care system and the white power and privilege which is embedded in its origins, its mission and purpose and its historic structures."[17]

The death of an AIDS activist in 2004 exemplified the points made by Barndt and highlighted the racial divide among patients with HIV/AIDS. Joseph Bostic ended up homeless and HIV-positive after spending seventeen years in prison. Then he changed his life, cofounding the New York City AIDS Housing Network for low-income people with HIV/AIDS. His income from this work, however, was minimal, and he had health insurance only some of the time. Likewise, he did not consistently take the expensive HIV medications.[18]

Bostic's death and that of another AIDS activist, Keith Cylar, at the same time led to reflections on AIDS in the African-American community. Although death rates from AIDS have dropped significantly since the new combination therapies, deaths among African-Americans have been proportionately much higher than for whites. "Among black men ages 25 to 44, the death rate from HIV/AIDS was more than six times greater than for whites. For black women in the same age group, the numbers are even more startling: the death rate is more than 13 times greater than for whites."[19]

A physician at Massachusetts General Hospital who has treated HIV/AIDS patients for twenty years, Dr. Valerie E. Stone, is especially alarmed about the death rates among African-Americans. "This epidemic is out of control in the black community."[20]

Researchers say this divide is due to late diagnoses and poorer care for African-Americans, who also have more complications because of other illnesses. These include hypertension, stroke, cardiovascular disease, and diabetes.

Dr. Joseph C. Gathe, Jr., a director of an AIDS clinic in Houston summarizes the situation this way: "the area my clinic's in is essentially a suburb of the third world. It's a shame no one seems to know that the problem in Africa looks like the problem in inner-city Houston, Chicago and New York."[21]

Dr. Daniel Kuritzkes, director of AIDS research at Brigham and Women's Hospital in Boston, expresses similar thoughts, describing two different and unequal tracks of HIV treatment in the United States. In the ideal path, a person is diagnosed as HIV-positive, gets medical care with regular follow-ups, and tolerates the regular regimen of medications. The expectation is for a fairly normal life. On the other track are those who come to the hospital having already developed AIDS. "They may have limited access to care because of finances or because other social or medical problems interfere. By and large, the deaths are among this group, which tends to be African-American."[22]

African-Americans have a shorter life expectancy than whites. Those who are HIV-positive are more likely to be uninsured or underinsured than whites. Studies have indicated that African-Americans receive lower-quality medical care, including less sophisticated treatments for HIV, even when money is not a factor.[23]

While the statistics are not as bad in the Hispanic community as in the African-American community, HIV/AIDS is still a grave problem, requiring attention and action. Many of the challenges are the same, though additional issues often include language barriers and (sometimes illegal) immigration for work and then returning to one's home country infected.

Besides confronting the long-term and immediate effects of racism, minorities who are infected must also face harmful dynamics in their own communities, such as homophobia, machismo, denial, and condemnations from religious leaders.[24]

OPPRESSION OF WOMEN

In our world almost half of all people living with HIV are female. Considerably more than half of the HIV-positive people in sub-Saharan Africa are women. In most areas, an increasing proportion of HIV-positive persons are women and girls. Young women aged fifteen to twenty-four are three times more likely to be infected than young men the same age.

The UNAIDS report on Women and AIDS moves beyond such statistics to highlight the profound and complex risks faced by women. "In reality, women and girls face a range of HIV-related risk factors and vulnerabilities that men and boys do not—many of which are embedded in the social relations and economic realities of their societies. These factors are not easily dislodged or altered, but until they are, efforts to contain and reverse the AIDS epidemic are unlikely to achieve sustained success."[25]

What are some of these factors? Unequal gender relations, unequal access to resources, poverty, violence, and sexual abuse profoundly limit women's freedom and put them at risk of infection. In many cultures and countries, women experience a subordinate status; men have sexual and economic power, supported by social norms and even laws. "Choosing to abstain or have safer sex is not an option for the millions of women around the world who endure rape and sexual violence."[26] Gillian Paterson explicitly expresses this reality:

> The powerlessness of many women when it comes to negotiating safe sex has been repeatedly stressed. . . . Abstinence? You don't become a mother, nor may you remain a wife for long, by abstaining. Monogamy? Many women are monogamous; they may be infected, without knowing it, by unfaithful or drug-injecting partners. Condoms? Just try persuading a man to use a condom when he doesn't want to. Negotiation with your partner? If cultural bias against open discussion of sexual matters co-exists with the cultural expectation that women are "innocent" in these matters, then how does either partner initiate such a discussion, let alone the female one?[27]

Women also face unequal property and inheritance rights, especially in South Asia and Africa where property is usually owned by men. A variety of laws and traditions have protected this practice.

> The payment of bride-price upon marriage tightens men's control over women and property . . . [and] reduces women's economic security and can lead to women having to endure abusive relationships or resort to sex for economic survival. . . . Lacking the enforceable right to own or inherit land and property, women and girls risk possible destitution after the death of their partners or parents, while poverty and economic dependence leave them exposed to increased sexual exploitation and violence.[28]

Another important aspect of the unequal access to resources is education. Studies show that education can bring some social power and employment opportunities to women, and so lower the risk of infection.[29] However, there is a large gap between education for boys and education for girls, a gap actually made worse by the AIDS epidemic (as was described in the earlier section on poverty). Access to knowledge, training, and technology is often determined along gender lines, discriminating against women.[30]

Education can also put young girls at risk, from male students or from teachers who demand sex for good grades. Another risk is that the young girl will use sex—often with older males—to earn money for school fees. Sex between young women and older men is common in many countries, even culturally valued. Nevertheless, the older men are more likely to be HIV-positive because of their multiple partners, and women, especially young girls, are biologically more susceptible to infection.

As Nsanga's story exemplified, a woman may also turn to sex as a way to support herself and her children. Lack of education, poverty, no income-earning opportunities, and male domination all blend together in a lethal mix.

Another example of access to resources is treatment and care. Voluntary counseling and testing services are much too scarce, even for pregnant women (to protect their newborn children). Some women refuse testing and treatment that are available for fear of violence and abandonment if their positive status becomes known.[31]

The burden of home-based care falls on women and girls. As the epidemic spreads, more women spend more time caring for infected family members. Girls may be forced to miss school or simply drop out entirely in order to help out. Income goes down, and problems increase. When the adult woman dies, the family may disintegrate, with children trying to parent their younger siblings or simply turning to life on the streets. Often a grandmother may become the caregiver. Some studies show that grandmothers are taking in many more orphans now than just ten years ago. Many times, of course, the burden becomes too great for this to happen.[32]

Previously we have already encountered the stories of several women: Shunila, DeShala Thompson, Lizzie Porter, and Nsanga.[33] Similar issues emerge in the experiences of these women and millions more around the globe. Poverty, lack of education, low social status, subordination, and little freedom are not just theories in U.N. reports but realities that undermine human flourishing and promote the spread of HIV/AIDS. For many women, injecting drug use, either by themselves and/or by their sexual partner, complicates the situation even more (risk of infected blood in shared needles, impairment of judgment about sex, and exchanging sex for drugs).

Such stories lead Paterson to describe the complex challenge concerning women in the time of AIDS.

> "The bleak reality," says WHO [the World Health Organization], "is that the sexual and economic subordination of women fuels the HIV pandemic." This view is supported by grassroots research and endorsed, now, by all responsible international agencies. Its implications are far-reaching. If a woman has no effective control over her own body, then it's no good expecting her to make responsible decisions about her sexuality. If she is poor, then long-term health risks may seem irrelevant in relation to her own or her family's survival. And this in turn explains why prevention strategies that are limited to "knowing the facts" and "becoming aware of the risk" have not succeeded. Where opportunities for transmission are embodied in the social and cultural organization of communities, then bringing about behavior change will require more than knowledge of the facts.[34]

In the midst of the crisis, Paterson finds hope that cultures and societies will recognize that subordination of women is actually threatening the community's life. Such insight can be nurtured by and lead to increased gender awareness and analysis. Biological differences are given, but gender differences are learned. From the moment of birth, each person internalizes the expectations that others have for a male or female and gradually begins to judge according to these expectations. Paterson adds "the really interesting thing is how *natural* the gender arrangements seem when you look at your own society."[35]

She gives some examples from her society in England. She can choose her husband, own a car, take an equal part in deciding about children, and inherit property. As we have seen in this text, other cultures have very different gender arrangements (that may surprise or upset us or simply be so different that they are hard to understand and appreciate).

Still, Paterson notes:

> There is almost no society on earth where you can become "gender-aware" without reaching two conclusions: first, that women are less

socially privileged than men; and second, that men are the ones with the economic, political and commercial power.[36]

Statistics, stories, and suffering may finally lead to a new awareness, to a change in the balance of power that is satisfactory to both sides, to survival. The immense weight of custom and religion, however, often make such change so very difficult. Survival, Paterson suggests, may be a sufficient counterweight. "For gender analysis, the crucial questions to be asked at every stage are: 'What about the women? Where are the women?' And maybe also: 'What will happen to the men?' "[37]

Her final question is a reminder that gender issues are just as important for men. "The cultural and social expectations that heighten women's risk of HIV also increase men's own vulnerability to infection. Many men are also trapped by cultural and social expectations (e.g. proving one's manhood by having multiple sexual partners) which deny them their full humanity and desires."[38]

Concretely, then, how can this fundamental change be promoted? Programs that focus only on women will ultimately fail because they do not address the power of men in so many societies. Two types of programs do offer hope. The first uses "participatory methodologies" in which "the research population itself defines the objectives, reflects on its own practices, defines the problems, suggests and implements solutions, and monitors the results."[39] People in gender-specific groups explore their needs and desires in their sexual lives and look at the cultural influences impacting their lives. Eventually, men and women meet together to create new norms.[40]

The second type of initiative attempts to form public policies that reduce the imbalance of power between women and men, providing opportunities for women in education, economics, and politics.[41]

GLOBALIZATION

The recent development of the complex and multifaceted process known as globalization has had a direct and indirect impact on the HIV/AIDS pandemic. Globalization has become a powerful economic, political, social, and cultural force that is praised and promoted by some and challenged and condemned by others.

In fact, globalization still evades easy definition. Those who see it as a positive process describe it as a growing integration of economies and societies around the world that is integral to sustainable development and has the potential to improve significantly the lives of all. Those who are suspicious about globalization, while recognizing its potential, see it as the domination of the powerful over the weak and so stress more the negative results: marginalization, environmental damage, loss of cultural diversity, and the widening gap between rich and poor.[42]

Globalization, then, is about relationships, about the "increases in the networks of global interdependence."[43] This growing global interdependence impacts the lives of communities and countries in a variety of ways, including (1) the economy and labor, (2) culture and politics, (3) poverty, (4) the environment, and (5) human dignity and the common good. All of these realities, of course, are connected to HIV/AIDS.

(1) One of the expressions of globalization easiest to see and experience is labor and the economy. "Neoliberal globalization" is a term frequently used to describe the dominant economic model, a model based on free markets and free trade. This neoliberal view stresses privatization, decreased regulation by governments, and the lowering of barriers to international trade.

This international trade is growing immensely, facilitated by technological advances in communication and transportation. There is now a global division of labor, offering greater efficiency, the elimination of scarcity, and higher standards of living for those newly employed in developing countries—all this according to the supporters of the dominant economic model. Opponents see sweatshops rather than higher standards of living, with a downward pressure on wages, exploitation in the factories, and increasing income inequality.[44]

(2) Increases in the networks of global interdependence can profoundly change traditional systems of meaning and living. "Fundamental cultural convictions about gender and family, the land and community are challenged by market-based values that promote individual accumulation and secularization. This brings cultural benefits to some, but also widespread loss of cultural identity to many."[45]

Globalization has also changed political systems, with sovereign nations having to deal with global financial institutions such as the World Bank and the International Monetary Fund (IMF).

With decreased government control over cross-border transactions regarding investment, debt and even immigration, national governments are in effect held hostage to the mobility of globalized capital. Governments today must be concerned about luring investments by offering tax breaks, tariff concessions and promising lower levels of environmental and safety regulation as well as social welfare provision. The summons to serve the common good of one's national community by supporting and participating in the structures of public authority is increasingly giving way before global pressures for competitiveness and the necessity of compromising goals such as equity, social security and justice in the domestic realm.[46]

(3) A central concern with globalization is poverty. Will this market economy really lead to prosperity for all, as supporters say?[47] Or will poverty actually increase? The UN's *Human Development Report* has indicated that the difference between rich and poor keeps on increasing and that a number of poor countries are getting even poorer.[48]

Although the World Bank and IMF were created to fight poverty and to promote a healthy world economy, some of their policies, rooted in the dominant neoliberal model, have actually had a harsh impact on many poor people in the developing world, for example, by demanding production for export rather than for local needs. This focus has contributed to increased hunger and malnutrition. Other pressures to meet debt payments have led to decreased budgets for education and health care.[49]

(4) Globalization's focus on market forces and maximization of profits puts the environment in grave danger. Free trade policies allow companies to relocate to countries with cheap labor and little protection for the laborer or the environment.[50]

Pope John Paul II expressed concerns about a wide range of environmental problems, including deforestation, water and air pollution, ozone depletion, and global warming. He stated that the "deterioration of the environment has been increasing rapidly. Indeed, the way resources are exploited must change as soon as possible."[51]

(5) Foundational to all these issues are human dignity and the common good. A slight paraphrase of the U.S. bishops' *Economic Justice for All* gets at the heart of this point: What does globalization do for people? What does it do to people? And how do people participate in it?

Those who support the neoliberal model of globalization claim that free trade policies will create wealth and provide opportunities for social development, a partial answer to the first question. Many critics of this model, in fact, claim that even that partial answer is not accurate (as indicated in the *Human Development Reports*). But even if it were, deeper questions must be asked: questions beyond markets and money and questions about the meaning and value of life.

What does this form of globalization do to people? Jesuit leaders from Latin America answered this question by stating that the logic of neoliberal globalization reduces "the greatness of man and woman to their capacity to generate monetary income. This intensifies individualism and the race to earn and to own, and easily leads to attacks on the integrity of creation. In many cases, greed, corruption, and violence are unleashed."[52] And so, communities are destroyed, and religious and cultural traditions are undermined by market-driven values.

John Paul II expressed his concern this way: "The market imposes its way of thinking and acting, and stamps its scale of values upon behavior. Those who are subjected to it often see globalization as a destructive flood threatening the social norms which had protected them and the cultural points of reference which had given them direction in life."[53] The vision of human dignity and the common good is lost in the emphasis on the individual.

And how do people participate in such globalization? Often by bearing the costs but usually not in decisions about international trade policies or labor and environmental conditions.

This very brief consideration of globalization reveals its impact on many dimensions of life in countries, communities, and individuals—and so on the spread of HIV/AIDS. To move from this more abstract discussion to the concrete details of real people, one only has to return again to Nsanga's story earlier in this chapter.

Already facing poverty, Nsanga and her family turn from a difficult life to face a tragic one when her husband loses his job as a schoolteacher. Marriage and family begin to unravel as a result of Zaire's national debt and the IMF's structural adjustment policies. The cutbacks in education and health care that came from budget pressures lead finally to death and the destruction of this family. Political and economic structures combine with already existing poverty, oppression of women, and lack of education to facilitate the growth of the AIDS pandemic.

Globalization has an even more direct connection with HIV/AIDS in the policies and practices of the major drug companies. The need for continuing research and development, patent laws, and international trade agreements conflict with poverty, the urgent need for antiretroviral drugs, and dying people. A profound and powerful conflict indeed!

Research-based pharmaceutical companies realistically need profits in order to continue innovation and the development of improved drugs (as well as a reward for the difficulties and risks). In the developed world, medications for HIV/AIDS remain very costly, far out of reach of developing countries and a huge percentage of HIV-positive persons. The result has been either a push to reduce the prices greatly for the sale of medications to the developing world or the production of generic drugs (versions of existing drugs) by companies in poor or middle-income countries, for example, India, China, or Brazil.[54]

The patent system, especially now in its globalized form, protects the investments and profits of the pharmaceutical companies. A key aspect of this system is the Trade Related Aspects of Intellectual Property Rights (TRIPS), approved in 1994. A country must accept TRIPS' rules on patents and copyrights in order to become a member of the World Trade Organization. There was an initial grace period that expired in 2005 (except for the poorest countries). Also, an exception allows countries not to follow TRIPS in a national emergency, either by purchasing medications in a country where the price is low and using it in a country where the price is high (this is called "parallel importation") or by ordering a patent holder to let generics be made in the country at risk (called "compulsory licensing"). In this situation, the original company receives a reasonable royalty, but the generic drives down the cost significantly.[55]

"Although compulsory licensing and parallel imports are legal under WTO rules, the U.S. government (through its trade representatives, who are heavily lobbied by the pharmaceutical industry) has often used its influence to attempt to dissuade poor countries from adopting these policies."[56] Also, PEPFAR initially refused to approve any generics for use in that program (though some have since been approved).

The major drug companies have entered into agreements with some developing countries to reduce greatly the prices of medications. In June 2005, for example, Bristol-Myers Squibb drastically cut the prices of two drugs for children in least developed countries (a generic form of one of these drugs was one of those approved by PEPFAR). At the same time Abbot Laboratories agreed with Brazil to reduce the cost of a drug for which Brazil had threatened to issue a compulsory license.[57]

Still, tensions and concerns remain. India had taken advantage of the "grace period" in TRIPS to produce generic versions of AIDS drugs for sale in many parts of the developing world (although India did not provide subsidized drugs to its own people[58] and although WHO removed some of these products from its preapproved list). In 2005, to satisfy the World Trade Organization's conditions, India revised its patent law restricting the production of generic medications.

Because so many countries had depended on the Indian products, treatment advocates worried about a crisis in available medications in the present and about "second line" antiretroviral therapies to respond to drug resistance in the future. Other AIDS researchers found hope in using compulsory licenses if necessary.[59]

AIDS activists acknowledge the pharmaceutical industry's political power and great profits but also claim that change to help the poor of the world is possible. They point out that "the industry's continued participation in AIDS drug work is indispensable,"[60] so cooperation is absolutely necessary. Among their recommendations for expanding access to AIDS treatment in the developing world are the following: (1) take advantage of possibilities built into TRIPS and pressure politicians to support this; (2) fully fund the Global Fund to Fight AIDS, TB and Malaria; (3) promote public-private partnerships; (4) develop differential pricing for medications sold in resource-rich and resource-poor countries; and (5) reevaluate the existing global intellectual property rights structures.[61]

Clearly, globalization directly impacts people's lives. Without a very large and stable supply of antiretroviral treatments (either generic or very low-cost originals), millions will die prematurely.

WAR AND OTHER VIOLENCE

Ethnic and religious conflicts, genocide, and the many forms of violence connected with wars are major contributors to the spread of HIV. Refugee camps have become perfect breeding grounds for HIV/AIDS. Rape is used as a weapon of war, not only as violence but as an attempt to destroy the bonds of family and community. Ironically, even the presence of peacekeeping forces leads to higher rates of HIV infection—and so eventually to death.

Wars, including numerous civil wars, have created millions of refugees, many of them women and children. All forms of forced migration, whether because of wars, economics, or natural disasters, lead to a breakdown of family and community, to a loss of cultural structures and norms, and to a lack of basic needs like food and shelter and education. "HIV flourishes, particularly, in situations of hopelessness and social breakdown. HIV control demands a measure of control over one's own life, a sense of self, of self-worth, and a belief that there is a future which is worth planning for. In a refugee camp, women and children have none of these."[62]

One tragic example in recent years of such a situation is Darfur, a western region of Sudan. As many as two million people have fled their homes to look for shelter in refugee camps. Not surprisingly they do not find sufficient food, water, or medicine. They do find unimaginable difficulties and dangers. "It is particularly difficult to monitor the health of internally displaced people, especially when their displacement is due to political factors, thus making their vulnerability to HIV infection or discrimination more acute."[63]

In countries with high levels of HIV and AIDS, HIV infection rates among the military are often significantly higher. Thus, the movement of troops, either for war or for peacekeeping, or for relief work, can lead to higher infection rates, for example, among sex workers. There is the additional risk of new viral strains being introduced in all the communities.[64]

A host of other threats are part of the vicious cycles of HIV/AIDS and social structures and dynamics related to war and its impact. Some are surprisingly practical—such as the location of water supplies or latrines in the refugee camps. If these locations are too isolated, young girls and boys and women who must go to these places face an increased risk of rape. Others are profoundly human—such as seeking sex as a source of affection. Also, in "post genocide situations, sex and the desire for pregnancy may become a means for replacing lost family, community and/or ethnic group."[65]

Others are related to issues already considered, for example, poverty and the oppression of women. In conflict situations and in emergencies following natural disasters, men are usually the decision-makers and the ones controlling resources. "Men usually control relief supplies and can barter these in exchange for women's only tradable commodity—sex."[66]

Other risky situations face health-care workers as they try to help others in the midst of conflict and emergency, often with very limited resources. Those receiving treatment for wounds may be HIV-positive; there may also be contaminated medical instruments.[67] Wars and other violence, of course, worsen the situations of those already suffering from AIDS, disrupting treatment and basic care. The newsletter of the African Jesuit AIDS Network describes one such situation in Burundi, where government forces and armed rebels continued fighting. A young Jesuit serving as the acting director of the AIDS Program in Bujumbura rejected the chance to be evacuated. Instead he helped other AIDS workers to provide supplies to two thousand refugees who had fled to the National Museum. They tried to visit some of the AIDS patients in the city hospitals and worried about "the survival of the very ill AIDS-sufferers who were too weak to flee the fighting."[68] After the fighting slowed down, the Jesuit AIDS Project resumed its usual activities of visits, care, and promoting prevention.

Wars and all the forms of violence linked to wars demand nuanced and sustained response to slow the spread of HIV/AIDS. Massive support and supplies need to be given to organizations attempting to meet immediate needs, such as UNICEF, Oxfam, and Doctors Without Borders. All of these persons themselves need to be attentive to promote and observe best practices to prevent the transmission of HIV. The role of the United Nations in addressing the endless conflicts must be strengthened in order to restore social and political stability. Participation by local groups, especially of women, in designing the distribution of humanitarian relief may help shift the power imbalances. "This will also help to ensure that the responses are culturally appropriate, realizable in practice and expressed in a language understood by those most affected."[69]

ETHICS

Given the complex, interwoven nature of these structural issues and given their immense impact on the spread of the AIDS pandemic, what response can the Consistent Ethic of Life make? Although this ethic was developed mainly in response to issues in the United States, from the very beginning war was one of those issues. Other themes in the Consistent Ethic of Life also apply directly to the structural issues of this chapter. With its roots in the Catholic Social Teachings, the Consistent Ethic of Life can begin its response by recognizing the sinfulness of some of these social structures.

Both Pope Paul VI and Pope John Paul II developed this idea. In his apostolic exhortation on the tenth anniversary of the closing of Vatican II, *Evangelization in the Modern World*, Paul VI proclaimed that evangelization includes an "explicit message . . . about life in society, about international life, peace, justice and development—a message especially today about liberation."[70] He also affirmed that liberation must be more than just politics or economics; it must be rooted in the gospel proclamation of Jesus. It requires conversion of structures and hearts.

Pope Paul VI developed what the Synod of Bishops had stated in 1971 about social structures that created problems. "There was a double understanding of the dynamic of personal and structural sin: human beings structure the sinfulness into a social system or arrangement, and the system or structure coercively shaped the behavior of individuals, both those who oppress and those who are oppressed."[71]

Pope John Paul II expressed a similar point in his 1987 encyclical *On Social Concern*: "one must denounce the existence of economic, financial and social *mechanisms* which, although they are manipulated by people, often function almost automatically, thus accentuating the situation of wealth for some and poverty for the rest."[72]

Later in the encyclical, John Paul II stressed that structures of sin are rooted in personal sin.[73] In this context he referred to an earlier exhortation in which he boldly described the sinners:

> It is a case of the very personal sins of those who cause or support evil or who exploit it; of those who are in a position to avoid, eliminate or at least limit certain social evils but who fail to do so out of laziness, fear or the conspiracy of silence, through secret complicity or indifference; of those who take refuge in the supposed impossibility of changing the world, and also of those who sidestep the effort and sacrifice required, producing specious reasons of a higher order.[74]

John Paul II also offered a path for overcoming the structures of sin. "It is above all a question of *interdependence*, sensed as a *system determining* relationships in the contemporary world, in its economic, cultural, political and religious elements, and accepted as a *moral category*."[75] Thus grows solidarity with its commitment to the common good. John Paul saw this solidarity as the path to authentic development and peace.[76]

Poverty, racism, oppression of women, some forms of globalization, and war and violence of all kinds destroy life, undermine human dignity, increase inequality, and divide the human family. These sinful social structures also facilitate the rapid spread of HIV/AIDS. A necessary dimension of the Consistent Ethic of Life's response, then, is the recognition of the structural nature of the pandemic and the willingness and courage to change these structures.[77]

Such change is grounded in basic convictions described in chapter 2. The life, teachings, and actions of Jesus model both care and compassion for individuals and also concern about oppressive structures of society. The healing of the leper gives a powerful example of both (see Mark 1:40–42 and chapter 2).

The Christian tradition built on Jesus's example, developed key principles and applied them in the social teachings. Human dignity, solidarity, justice, and the universal common good offer a solid foundation for recognizing and changing sinful social structures. This Christian vision of the value and interdependence of all creation, especially human beings, contrasts with the emphasis on rights in the United States' tradition. This tradition protects individual rights from outside abuse, but the Christian vision establishes a positive obligation to help others. The focus and energy are in opposite directions. As a result, the Christian vision leans on the U.S. tradition to do more, to help create right relationships along with the structural recognition of the human dignity and rights and responsibilities of all people. Economic and political structures that oppress are clearly evil. Charity is important but not sufficient. Justice must also flourish.

According to the social teachings, a central aspect of this good society is the recognition that the goods of this world are meant for all. This conviction, rooted in the belief that the goods of the earth were created by God to be shared by all, is called "the universal destination of goods." It places significant limits on the right to private property and so to corporations' structures to maximize profits. "Private property, in fact, is under a 'social mortgage,' which means that it has an intrinsically social function, based upon and justified precisely by the principle of the universal destination of goods."[78]

John Paul II went on to name a number of areas where reforms according to this principle are urgently needed. (His words also address directly some of the concerns of this chapter.)

> In this respect I wish to mention specifically: the reform of the international trade system, which is mortgaged to protectionism and increasing bilateralism; the reform of the world monetary and financial

system, today recognized as inadequate; the question of technological exchanges and their proper use; the need for a review of the structure of the existing International Organizations, in the framework of an international juridical order. . . .

The existing Institutions and Organizations have worked well for the benefit of peoples. Nevertheless, humanity today is in a new and more difficult phase of its genuine development. It needs a greater degree of international ordering, at the service of the societies, economies and cultures of the whole world.[79]

The Consistent Ethic of Life, of course, incorporates these values and principles from Scripture and Tradition. Other themes expressed in the Consistent Ethic can also enrich and give guidance for recognizing and changing sinful social structures that facilitate the growth of the HIV/AIDS epidemic. Some of these themes are the preferential option for the poor, the feminization of poverty, the use of limited resources, the growing appreciation of nonviolence, and the need for dialogue.

While discussing the U.S. bishops' pastoral letter on economic justice, Cardinal Bernardin highlighted the Church's preferential option for the poor. He noted that this concept is rooted in the Scriptures, was creatively developed by theologians in Latin America, and has now become an important dimension of Church teaching. The preferential option for the poor "calls the Church to speak for the poor, to see the world from their perspective, and to empty itself so it may experience the power of God in the midst of poverty and powerlessness."[80]

Cardinal Bernardin acknowledged how challenging this concept is for the Church's mission and ministry. He named two ways in which the Church has attempted to respond to poverty. The first—and better known—is the Church's direct service to the poor through hospitals, orphanages, and shelters. The second—and more controversial—is the Church's role "as advocate and actor in the public life of society."[81] This role leads the Church to evaluate social and economic structures in light of social justice and to encourage and take action to help create a society of solidarity, justice, and peace.[82]

Previous sections of this book have described many examples of the urgent need for both expressions of the preferential option for the poor in the context of HIV and AIDS.

A particular dimension of poverty is its impact on women. Another popular phrase captures this harsh reality: the feminization of poverty.

First used in the context of poverty and women in the United States, this concept helps to focus attention on the situation of women around the world. The statistics and the stories of the women in this book exemplify the necessity of such focus—and action to change the structures that oppress women.

In his address Cardinal Bernardin emphasized that standing with the most vulnerable in the world demands more than fine rhetoric. It demands both direct social services and systemic structures and programs. In the U.S. context, Cardinal Bernardin mentioned child care and food stamps and aid to families with children. Not these specific programs necessarily but programs like them are "a fundamental requirement of a just society."[83]

Another aspect of the option for the poor is the use of limited resources. Cardinal Bernardin actually raised this issue in the context of health care, though with a specific look at the United States. The fundamental insights, however, easily translate into the discussion of treatment for HIV and AIDS throughout the world.

Addressing the lack of health care available to so many of the poor in the United States, Cardinal Bernardin stated:

> A serious problem today is the fact that many persons are left without basic health care while large sums of money are invested in the treatment of a few by means of exceptional, expensive measures. While technology has provided the industry with many diagnostic and therapeutic tools, their inaccessibility, cost and sophistication often prevent their wide distribution and use.[84]

He then added "many persons do not and probably will not receive the kind of basic care that nurtures life—unless we change attitudes, policies and programs."[85] He suggested some concrete practices to express the Consistent Ethic of Life in Catholic health-care institutions, such as practices that challenge the usual way of business and practices that boldly serve the needs of the poor. For example, not transferring a patient to a state institution when the person's insurance runs out.[86]

A link between the theme of scarce resources and that of nonviolence is found in the production and sale of weapons of war. Already in Vatican II's "The Church in the Modern World," the bishops of the world stated:

Rather than eliminating the causes of war, the arms race serves only to aggravate the position. As long as extravagant sums of money are poured into the development of new weapons, it is impossible to devote adequate aid in tackling the misery which prevails at the present day in the world. Instead of eradicating international conflict once and for all, the contagion is spreading to other parts of the world. . . . Therefore, we declare once again: the arms race is one of the greatest curses on the human race and the harm it inflicts on the poor is more than can be endured.[87]

In his 1993 address commemorating the tenth anniversary of the U.S. bishops' pastoral letter *The Challenge of Peace*, Cardinal Bernardin expressed a similar conviction. "Diverting scarce resources away from the purchase of arms to meeting basic human needs for food, shelter, education, and health care would go a long way toward building a just and peaceful world."[88]

Pope John Paul II's increasing emphasis on nonviolence, especially as expressed in his messages for World Peace Day, undoubtedly influenced a similar focus in the Consistent Ethic of Life.[89] However, already in 1985, Cardinal Bernardin challenged the conviction that society must meet violence with violence. As a result, he rejected capital punishment as an appropriate response to crime, as a way to protect society. He asserted that violence is not the way to break the cycle of violence.

We desperately need an attitude or atmosphere in society which will sustain a consistent defense and promotion of life. Where human life is considered "cheap" and easily "wasted," eventually nothing is held as sacred and all lives are in jeopardy. The purpose of proposing a consistent ethic of life is to argue that success on any one of the issues threatening life requires a concern for the broader attitude in society about respect for life. Attitude is the place to root an ethic of life. Change of attitude, in turn, can lead to change of policies and practices in our society.[90]

In order to connect the Consistent Ethic of Life to public policy, Cardinal Bernardin recognized the need for frequent dialogue with others. Of course, dialogue is necessary for the proper development of the life ethic itself, benefiting from various perspectives in order to arrive at a better appreciation of truth. Dialogue is also necessary to find appropriate expressions in a pluralistic world. Not everyone will share the same convictions of faith but may find other common ground. Dialogue implies "that one person or one church or one scholarly community or one think tank" does not have all the answers.[91]

In a later address Cardinal Bernardin urged the Church to "resist the sectarian tendency to retreat into a closed circle, convinced of our truth and the impossibility of sharing it with others. To be both prophetic and public, a countersign to much of the culture, but also a light and leaven for all of it, is the delicate balance to which we are called."[92]

The Church, Bernardin said, can both teach the world and learn much from it. "A confident Church will speak its mind, seek as a community to live its convictions, but leave space for others to speak to us, help us to grow from their perspective, and to collaborate with them."[93]

Moving from theory to practice, of course, is almost always very challenging, and it is especially so in the complexity and suffering of the AIDS epidemic. Still, human dignity, solidarity, justice, and the universal common good provide profound and solid ethical foundations for life-respecting and life-saving practices. The preferential option for the poor, the recognition of the feminization of poverty, the just use of scarce resources, the growing appreciation of nonviolence, and the need for dialogue offer concrete alternatives to sinful social structures.

What specific actions might spring from this Consistent Ethic of Life? What links can we establish between this ethical vision and the social, political, and economic policies and practices that promote the transmission of HIV?

We have already seen examples of the vicious cycles of economic policies, poverty, and the oppression of women and the dehumanization and death these cycles cause. Breaking into a vicious cycle is so very difficult; it seems that many actions must be taken simultaneously.[94]

Certainly, though, one key entry point is the crushing poverty experienced by so many millions of people in our world. At the structural level, a number of changes are possible. One of those changes, the relief of some international debt, has already begun. To celebrate the new millennium, many groups and individuals (including Pope John Paul II) urged the forgiveness of massive debts of some of the poorest nations. These debts, often encouraged by international institutions and incurred by corrupt leaders, continue to oppress the debtor nations, limiting and reducing health care and education. More debt forgiveness along with responsible use of their resources by local governments will further reduce poverty, promote the common good, and address AIDS directly.[95]

One practice that greatly increased debts was the purchase of weapons. So arms sales promotes both violence and poverty. Changing that dynamic would offer a double benefit, reducing violence and having funds to address some of the root causes of conflict and disease.[96]

Another possible economic change is the creation of free trade agreements that are fair, especially for the poor. Fair agreements will be aware of the perspective of the poor and not just the powerful.[97] The preferential option for the poor will probably not convince many leaders of governments and corporations, but demonstrations that ethical business practices are ultimately also good business practices might. Another motivation is security, as poverty nourishes not only HIV/AIDS but also terrorism. Both the possibility of seeing the world from the side of the poor and the need for different motivations and values highlight the central place for dialogue if change is to occur.

One attempt to facilitate such dialogue is Open Space.

> Open Space works best when the work to be done is complex, the people and ideas involved are diverse, the passion for resolution (and potential for conflict) are high, and the time to get it done was yesterday. It's been called passion bounded by responsibility, the energy of a good coffee break, intentional self-organization, spirit at work, chaos and creativity, evolution in organization, and a simple, powerful way to get people and organizations moving—when and where it's needed most.[98]

Surely changing the sinful social structures that promote the HIV/AIDS pandemic is where it is needed most!

When dialogue fails or is not even attempted, advocacy and activism may be necessary to achieve change. Such pressure best reflects the Consistent Ethic of Life when it is nonviolent. One example of surprising success of such advocacy has been some of the changes accepted by the major pharmaceutical companies.[99]

Publicizing the success of nonviolent resistance and advocacy is essential. Many people instinctively slip into the age-old conviction (indeed, religion) that only violence saves. The success of nonviolence, especially in recent years, must be recognized and taught so that new attitudes may develop.[100]

Almost always, groups, large or small, will be needed to change social and economic structures. While some people find hope in the promise and work of small faith communities to effect these changes, others point to the pervasive influence of such structures and so recognize the need for the involvement of corporations and governments and media.

Although institutions have their own interiority and spirituality,[101] individuals both contribute to and can change these institutions. What can individuals do regarding sinful social structures? Individuals can begin by accepting responsibility to change their worldview by moving beyond many messages from their own societies to acknowledge the reality of economic and political policies and practices that oppress people. Such insight often comes from experience rather than from mere words, from contact not just concepts.[102]

Such insight leads to some kind of action. Some individuals may choose to volunteer for several years to participate with international groups attempting to meet immediate needs and to plant seeds for structural change, for example, Peace Corps or Jesuit Volunteers International. Others may choose a career with the Centers for Disease Control and Prevention, Bread for the World, or Doctors Without Borders. Still others may support such organizations with their donations.

Individuals may donate their time to advocacy groups. Surely not all aspects of the vicious cycles can be addressed by one group, but a part can be. Groups based in parishes or schools can inform others about sweatshops and promote alternative fair-trade goods. Other individuals can participate in groups addressing racism or family violence or inferior education in their cities.

Individuals can become directors of corporations and create more just policies. At lower levels similar choices and practices can be implemented. Other individuals can work to enhance corporate responsibility through shareholder resolutions.

Individuals can vote, choosing candidates that challenge sinful structures and create alternatives. Individuals can name and critique antilife aspects of the political parties. Individuals can run for office.

Individuals can try to live authentically the Consistent Ethic of Life in all dimensions of their lives.

NOTES

1. John Paul II, *The Gospel of Life* (Boston: Pauline Books & Media, 1995), 26 (para. 12).

2. Ann Smith and Enda McDonagh, *The Reality of AIDS* (Maynooth, Ireland: Trocaire, Veritas, CAFOD, 2003), 6.

3. Smith and McDonagh, *Reality of AIDS*, 26.

4. Smith and McDonagh, *Reality of AIDS*, 26–28.

5. Nsanga's story is taken from Brooke Grundfest Schoepf, "Health, Gender Relations, and Poverty in the AIDS Era," in *Courtyards, Markets, City Streets: Urban Women in Africa*, ed. Kathleen Sheldon (Boulder, Colo.: Westview Press, 1996), 153–68.

6. Schoepf, "Health, Gender Relations," 157–58.

7. Schoepf, "Health, Gender Relations," 159.

8. Schoepf, "Health, Gender Relations," 160.

9. Schoepf, "Health, Gender Relations," 166.

10. Schoepf, "Health, Gender Relations," 167.

11. Dahleen Glanton, "Emerging Face of HIV," *Chicago Tribune*, 28 March 2004, 1.

12. Joseph R. Barndt, "The Interrelationship of Racism and AIDS," *Council of Religious AIDS Networks*, www.aidsfaith.com/convocation/paperidx.asp (accessed 11 July 2005).

13. Barndt, "Interrelationship."

14. Barndt, "Interrelationship."

15. Barndt, "Interrelationship."

16. Barndt, "Interrelationship."

17. Barndt, "Interrelationship."

18. Linda Villarosa, "Patients with H.I.V. Seen as Separated by a Racial Divide," *New York Times*, 7 August 2004 (can be found at www.natap.org/2004/HIV/080904_03.htm).

19. Villarosa, "Patients."

20. Villarosa, "Patients."

21. Villarosa, "Patients."

22. Villarosa, "Patients."

23. Villarosa, "Patients."

24. Read about the helpful work of the Balm in Gilead at www.balmingilead.org.

25. UNAIDS and WHO, "Women and AIDS: An Extract from the *AIDS Epidemic Update 2004*," *UNAIDS*, www.unaids.org/en/default.asp, then use search for title (accessed 12 July 2005), 4.

26. UNAIDS and WHO, "Women and AIDS," 7.

27. Gillian Paterson, *Women in the Time of AIDS* (Maryknoll, N.Y.: Orbis Books, 1996), 77.

28. UNAIDS and WHO, "Women and AIDS," 11.

29. UNAIDS and WHO, "Women and AIDS," 7.

30. UNAIDS and WHO, "Women and AIDS," 9.

31. UNAIDS and WHO, "Women and AIDS," 8.

32. UNAIDS and WHO, "Women and AIDS," 32.

33. It may be helpful to reread their stories at this point: Shunila, DeShala Thompson, and Lizzie Porter were discussed in chapter 4, and Nsanga is discussed earlier in this chapter.

34. Paterson, *Women in the Time*, xi–xii.

35. Paterson, *Women in the Time*, 31.

36. Paterson, *Women in the Time*, 31.

37. Paterson, *Women in the Time*, 33.

38. Smith and McDonagh, *Reality of AIDS*, 103.

39. Paterson, *Women in the Time*, xii.

40. Smith and McDonagh, *Reality of AIDS*, 106–7.

41. Smith and McDonagh, *Reality of AIDS*, 107–8.

42. Michael Czerny, S.J., "University and Globalization: Yes, But," *Santa Clara Lectures*, vol. 9, no. 1 (7 November 2002): 7–8.

43. Thomas Massaro, S.J., "Judging the Juggernaut: Toward an Ethical Evaluation of Globalization," *Blueprint for Social Justice*, vol. LVI, no. 1 (September 2002): 2.

44. Massaro, S.J., "Juggernaut," 2–3.

45. Czerny, S.J., "University," 5.

46. Massaro, S.J., "Juggernaut," 3.

47. See the writings of George Weigel, Richard Neuhaus, and Michael Novak; for example, Michael Novak, *The Catholic Ethic and the Spirit of Capitalism* (New York: Free Press, 1993).

48. Kevin Watkins, et al., "Human Development Report 2005," *United Nations Development Programme*, hdr.undp.org/reports/global/2005/pdf/HDR05_frontmatter.pdf (accessed 25 November 2005).

49. See Jim Yong Kim, Joyce Millen, Alec Irwin, and John Gershman, eds., *Dying for Growth: Global Inequality and the Health of the Poor* (Monroe, Me.: Common Courage, 2000).

50. See John Cavanaugh, et al, *Alternatives to Economic Globalization: A Better World Is Possible* (San Francisco: Berrett-Koehler, 2002).

51. John Paul II, "Is Liberal Capitalism the Only Path?" *Origins*, vol. 20, no. 2 (24 May 1990): 20; see also John Paul II's *The Ecological Crisis: A Common Responsibility*.

52. Jesuit Provincials of Latin America, "For Life and Against Neoliberalism," in *We Make the Road by Walking: Central America, Mexico, and the Caribbean in the New Millennium*, eds. Ann Butwell, Kathy Ogle, and Scott Wright (Washington: EPICA, 1998), 76.

53. John Paul II, "Address of the Holy Father to the Pontifical Academy of Social Sciences" *Holy See* www.vatican.va/holy_father/john_paul-ii/speeches/2001/documents/hf_jp-ii_spe_20010427_pc-social-sciences_en.html (accessed 14 July 2005).

54. These alternatives raise concerns about the quality of generic AIDS treatments and about the reimportation of generic/cut-cost drugs back into the United States. For thoughts on good ethics being good business, see Kevin O'Brien, S.J., and Peter Clark, S.J., "Drug Companies and AIDS in Africa," *America*, vol. 187, no. 17 (25 November 2002): 8–11.

55. Alexander Irwin, Joyce Millen, and Dorothy Fallows, *Global AIDS: Myths and Facts* (Cambridge, Mass.: South End Press, 2003), 116–22.

56. Irwin, Millen, and Fallows, *Global AIDS*, 122.

57. Keith Alcorn, "Brazil Reaches 11th Hour Deal on Drug Patent," *NAM*, www.aidsmap.com/en/news/83C0EF16-F9EC-4A9C-8200-5E07E99CB38D .asp (accessed 15 July 2005).

58. Irwin, Millen, and Fallows, *Global AIDS*, 120.

59. HDN Key Correspondent Team, "India, China or Brazil—Who Will Produce the Second Line ARVs?" *NAM*, www.aidsmap.com/en/news /24B33FA6-89CB-42BA-880F-18D774FF85D6.asp (accessed 15 July 2005).

60. Irwin, Millen, and Fallows, *Global AIDS*, 129.

61. Irwin, Millen, and Fallows, *Global AIDS*, 129–33.

62. Paterson, *Women in the Time*, 8.

63. Smith and McDonagh, *Reality of AIDS*, 113.

64. Smith and McDonagh, *Reality of AIDS*, 113–14.

65. Smith and McDonagh, *Reality of AIDS*, 117.

66. Smith and McDonagh, *Reality of AIDS*, 117.

67. Smith and McDonagh, *Reality of AIDS*, 115 and 118.

68. Florentino Badial, S.J., "AIDS in Time of War," from *AJA News* on 25 August 2003, ajanews@jesuits.ca (28 August 2003).

69. Smith and McDonagh, *Reality of AIDS*, 116.

70. Pope Paul VI, *Evangelization in the Modern World* (Washington: USCC Office of Publishing Services, 1976), 20.

71. Fred Kammer, S.J., *Doing Faithjustice* (Mahwah, N.J.: Paulist Press, 1991), 101–2.

72. Pope John Paul II, *On Social Concern* (Washington: USCC Office of Publishing Services, 1988), 16.

73. John Paul II, *Social Concern*, 36.

74. John Paul II, *Social Concern*, 36, footnote 65.

75. John Paul II, *Social Concern*, 38.

76. John Paul II, *Social Concern*, 39.

77. Kammer, *Faithjustice*, 161–88.

78. John Paul II, *Social Concern*, 42.

79. John Paul II, *Social Concern*, 43.

80. Joseph Cardinal Bernardin, "The Face of Poverty Today," in *Consistent Ethic of Life* (Kansas City: Sheed & Ward, 1988), 40.

81. Bernardin, "Poverty Today," 41.

82. Kammer, *Faithjustice*, 121–60.

83. Bernardin, "Poverty Today," 47.

84. Bernardin, "The Consistent Ethic of Life and Health Care Systems," in *Consistent Ethic*, 55.

85. Bernardin, "Health Care," 55.

86. Bernardin, "Health Care," 57.

87. Austin Flannery, O.P., ed., "Pastoral Constitution on the Church in the Modern World," in *Vatican Council II* (Northport, N.Y.: Costello Publishing Company, 1996), 81.

88. Joseph Cardinal Bernardin, "The Challenge of Peace—1993," in *A Moral Vision for America* (Washington, D.C.: Georgetown University Press, 1998), 100.

89. See, for example, the bishops' reflection *The Harvest of Justice Is Sown in Peace* (Washington, D.C.: USCCB Publishing, 1994).

90. Bernardin, "The Death Penalty in Our Time," in *Consistent Ethic*, 65.

91. Bernardin, "Role of the Religious Leader in the Development of Public Policy," in *Moral Vision*, 34.

92. Bernardin, "The Consistent Ethic of Life after Webster," in *Moral Vision*, 92.

93. Bernardin, "Webster," 92.

94. Kammer, *Faithjustice*, 189–204.

95. UNAIDS, "Debt-for-AIDS Swaps," *UNAIDS*, www.unaids.org/en/default.asp, then use search for title (accessed 20 July 2005); see also " 'Forgive and Forget' Won't Fix Third World Debt," *Worldwatch Institute*, www.worldwatch.org/press/news/2001/04/261.

96. William D. Hartung and Frida Berrigan, "Militarization of U.S. African Policy, 2000 to 2005," *World Policy Institute*, www.worldpolicy.org/projects/arms/reports.html (accessed 21 July 2005); see other reports at this same site; also, on this issue and others in this section, see Bishop William Skylstad, "Letter to President Bush: The G-8 Summit," *Origins*, vol. 35, no. 8 (7 July 2005).

97. See the statement by Central American and U.S. bishops on CAFTA at www.wola.org/economic/econ_trade.htm (accessed 22 July 2005); other information and statements from a human rights perspective can also be found there (Washington Office on Latin America).

98. Open Space, "About Open Space," *Worldwide Open Space*, www.openspaceworld.org/wiki/wiki/wiki.cgi?AboutOpenSpace (accessed 25 July 2005); for use of Open Space Technology in Haiti, see www.beyondborders.net; also see www.theworldcafe.com.

99. Irwin, Millen, and Fallows, *Global AIDS*, 115–33.

100. Walter Wink, *Engaging the Powers*, (Minneapolis: Fortress Press, 1992), 13–31 and 243–57.

101. Walter Wink, *The Powers That Be*, (New York: Doubleday, 1998), 1–11.

102. Peter-Hans Kolvenbach, S.J., "The Service of Faith and the Promotion of Justice in American Jesuit Higher Education," *Santa Clara University*, www.scu.edu/ignatiancenter/bannan/eventsandconferences/lectures/archives/kolvenbach.cfm (accessed 29 July 2005).

Chapter Eight

Creating the Future

HIV and AIDS raise ethical questions that extend throughout the life cycle and around the globe. In the previous chapters we have considered the guidance offered by the Consistent Ethic of Life for responding specifically to these questions. In this chapter we will locate these responses in the larger process of creating the future. With the emphasis on human experience and religious tradition, chapters 1 and 2 have already reminded us that this process has old roots and must continue to develop now.

In this chapter, then, we will follow three stages that cycle around and through the lives of individuals and communities: (1) lament, (2) action, and (3) trust in God.

LAMENT

Enter our lament in your book; store every tear in your flask (see Psalm 56). Earlier chapters have presented statistics and stories of intense and staggering suffering throughout the world. Suffering surrounds us—and has always confronted the human family. For thousands of years people have been searching for some meaning in suffering and have been asking "Why?" In the Bible, Job wrestled with suffering and with God. The early Christian community struggled to make sense of the horrible torture and execution of Jesus. Theologians have tried to hold suffering together with God's power, justice, love—and human freedom. (For more on this search, see appendix I.)

Yet, for all the struggle and searching, no simple answer has been found. Instead of leading to answers, overwhelming suffering leads spontaneously and appropriately to lament. "O Lord, I cry out to you. I am desperate." For most if not all of us, there are times in our lives when we want to join the Psalmist in crying out to God, expressing our despair and anger. Yet, we may hesitate, somehow sensing that we ought not address God in this way.

Fortunately, the Scriptures are rich in lament, teaching us that it is not only good but necessary to cry out to God. See, for example, the books of Job and Lamentations and also many of the Psalms, including 39, 44, 53, 77, 88, 89, 106, 109, and 143. Biblical scholars have helped us to appreciate what these laments meant to the people of God then[1] and what they can mean for us today.

Lament marked the very beginning of the history of the Hebrew people—and so the beginning of the Christian religious story, too. In their oppression the people cried out to God, and God heard and acted, leading them to freedom (see Exodus 2:23–25).

Lament is necessary for individuals. We all experience suffering in our lives: sickness, poverty, abuse, alienation, drugs, violence, and death. As we have seen in the previous chapters, HIV and AIDS often involve all these forms of suffering and more. People directly experiencing such intense suffering surely need to lament. So must others, overcoming their numbness and acknowledging the disease and death that affect so many millions of members of the human family.

Things are not right. The first step to grief and healing is to move from overwhelmed silence to speech, the bold speech of lament. The Psalms show us how to speak out against suffering and oppression, even against God. But such crying out allows us both to grieve and to grow into a mature covenant partner with God and not merely a subservient one.

Scripture scholar Walter Wink suggests a haunting image: "We human beings are far too frail and tiny to bear all this pain. What we need is a portable form of the Wailing Wall in Jerusalem, where we can unburden ourselves of this accumulated suffering. We need to experience it; it is part of reality. . . . We are to articulate these agonizing longings and let them pass through us to God."[2]

Lament is also necessary for life in society, raising questions of justice and power. The HIV/AIDS pandemic cannot be understood or addressed properly unless we appreciate the global structural issues described in chapter 7. Even lament has systemic implications. Another Scripture scholar, Walter Brueggemann, writes strongly: "For the managers of the system—political, economic, religious, moral—there is always a hope that the troubled folks will not notice the dysfunction or that a tolerance of a certain degree of dysfunction can be accepted as normal and necessary, even if unpleasant. Lament occurs when the dysfunction reaches an unacceptable level, when the injustice is intolerable and change is insisted upon."[3]

He adds that when lament is not allowed, justice questions gradually become ignored. When this happens, we miss the public systemic issues about which "biblical faith is relentlessly concerned."[4]

Lament allows us to move from silence to speech, from meditation to active hope. It renews and deepens our relationship with God, even as it questions and challenges God. Lament confronts the evils in our lives and religion and culture and world, proclaiming that these must not be.

ACTION

This is the fast that I wish: untying the thongs of the yoke, sharing your bread, not turning your back (see Isaiah 58:5–7). Lament leads to action. Throughout this book, we have considered many attempts to live the Consistent Ethic of Life, from very personal actions concerning life itself and the relationships of life to the actions of corporations and governments that shape our global society. Chapter 2 offered both religious models and motivation and directions for these actions. The prophets and Jesus all embody a faith that does justice and express a passionate concern for the poor and oppressed, including widows, orphans, and lepers.

The earlier chapters have indicated how such compassion and justice must be implemented in response to HIV and AIDS in the twenty-first century. The following are some examples of this. (1) Individuals can find sound direction in forming their conscience about respect for life in its beginnings and its endings in the long Christian tradition, including Vatican II's emphasis on the whole person understood in historical context. (2) In the face of overwhelming suffering, what is necessary is compassionate care and loving presence, not mercy killing. (3) Economic issues demand attention. Pregnant women must have greater access to treatment for their own health and for the health of their babies. Millions of orphans cry out for immediate help; resource-rich countries must hear this cry of the poor. (4) Individuals and communities must take responsibility to discern the social and cultural influences that promote irresponsibility, especially those that support male domination. (5) Government and transnational organizations must transform political and economic policies and structures that undermine human flourishing through violence and poverty.

Thus, the Consistent Ethic of Life offers sound guidance for creating the future.

The writings of Brueggemann and Wink also offer keen insight into creating the future with our actions. In his *The Prophetic Imagination*, Brueggemann emphasizes the need for imagination, the capacity to move from the wisdom and courage of the prophetic text to the new actual situation. Only then can one hope to effect "change in social perspective and social policy."[5]

The prophetic role, then, must embody and express both criticizing the oppressive social policy and energizing a despairing people. Lament, as mentioned earlier, is the beginning of radical criticism. It brings to public expression the fears and terrors that numbness has covered over. Those in power intuitively know that deception and oppression will collapse when this happens. "The riddle and insight of biblical faith is the awareness that only anguish leads to life, only grieving leads to joy, and only embraced endings permit new beginnings."[6]

The prophet's other role, then, is to help energize the people with hope. Brueggemann states, "Hope is the refusal to accept the reading of reality which is the majority opinion, and one does that only at great political and existential risk."[7] Therefore, hope is subversive. Brueggemann adds that hope is not optimism but is about a "covenant between a personal God and a community. Promise belongs to the world of trusting speech and faithful listening."[8]

As earlier chapters made so very clear, HIV and AIDS lead not only to overwhelming suffering but also to numbness. The pandemic's spread is fostered by oppressive political, economic, and social structures. The need for prophets with criticizing and energizing imagination is urgent.

Walter Wink has written extensively about the "principalities and powers."[9] He translates these biblical images into the present by interpreting them as the spirituality at the center of economic, social, and political institutions. "In the biblical view the Powers are at one and the same time visible *and* invisible, earthly *and* heavenly, spiritual *and* institutional (Col 1:15–20)."[10] Powers have physical manifestations (like buildings and personnel) along with an inner spirituality.

Wink asserts, with ample evidence, that the Powers have become evil, the institutions and systems have become integrated around "idolatrous values."[11] In this context, he asks a haunting question: "How can we oppose evil without creating new evils and being made evil ourselves?"[12]

Wink's conclusion is significant: "If we want to change those systems, we will have to address not only their outer forms, but their inner spirit as well."[13] Because unjust systems use institutionalized violence to perpetuate themselves, we too will be tempted to use violence. Then, of course, we too become trapped in violence, for "evil is contagious."[14] The way out, Wink offers, is to follow the nonviolent path of Jesus.[15]

Wink's understanding of the Powers at work in our world presents a remarkable framework for recognizing the many structural issues in the AIDS epidemic (see especially chapters 6 and 7) and for developing strategies for nonviolent change. The convictions and insights of the Consistent Ethic of Life and of the prophetic imagination can help transform the Powers and so create a better future.

Wisdom, of course, comes from many sources. UNAIDS has also looked to the future, specifically concerning AIDS in Africa. In this remarkable effort, three scenarios were created covering the years from the present until 2025. "The decisions we make about the future are guided by our view of how the world works and what we think is possible. A scenario is a story that describes a possible future. Building and using scenarios can help people and organizations to learn, to create wider and more shared understanding, to improve decision-making and to galvanise commitment and informed action."[16]

The scenarios include the religious perspectives of believers from many faiths along with the commitment to human rights of all concerned people. At the same time, the authors note that scenarios can be used to challenge assumptions and beliefs and to stretch worldviews, perhaps leading to new, creative action, action that many can take part in.[17]

In creating the three scenarios, the authors carefully considered five powerful forces that impact the spread of HIV/AIDS (all of these forces have been discussed in various ways in the earlier chapters of this book). The interaction of these forces, operating from the individual to the international, will determine the future of the pandemic.

The five "critical and uncertain forces" are (1) the growth or erosion of unity and integration: solidarity or factionalism will produce dramatically different levels of care and prevention; (2) the evolution of beliefs, values, and meanings: convictions about life and sexuality and illness and morality will emphasize stigma or compassion; (3) the leveraging of resources and capabilities: the best use of limited resources (both financial and human) must begin now; (4) the generation and application of knowledge: combining traditional and modern views of the world will be necessary to reach the greatest number of people; and (5) the distribution of power and authority: critical dimensions of this force will include gender, age, and the sharing (or centralization) of power.[18]

The first scenario, "Traps and Legacies," describes a future based on current trends. This is a story "in which Africa as a whole fails to escape from its more negative legacies, and AIDS deepens the traps of poverty, underdevelopment, and marginalization in a globalizing world."[19]

The second scenario, "Tough Choices," applies the dynamics of the most successful response presently developed. This is a story "in which African leaders choose to take tough measures that reduce the spread of HIV in the long term, even if it means difficulties in the short term."[20] There is future growth and development in Africa, though the pandemic will get worse before the situation gradually improves.

The third and most optimistic scenario, "Times of Transition," describes the impact of a comprehensive prevention and treatment program that is begun as quickly as possible. This is a story that shows what "might happen if all of today's good intentions were translated into the coherent and integrated development response necessary to tackle HIV and AIDS in Africa."[21]

What actions will result in this more positive outcome? The scenario includes the following: 1) rapid rollout of treatment and prevention programs; 2) national efforts to reduce poverty; 3) improved cooperation between Africa and international partners; 4) changes in global trade and in gender relations; and 5) the promotion of peace and security.[22]

Creating a better future is possible. *AIDS in Africa: Three Scenarios to 2025* is both realistic and challenging. The authors acknowledge that the death toll will rise no matter what is done and that Africa will continue to face major challenges. Creating a better future, they claim, will demand sufficient political will to change behavior, including the behavior of individuals and communities and institutions. People can choose to change or stop the forces driving the AIDS epidemic.[23]

TRUST IN GOD

Do not let your hearts be troubled; trust in God (see John 14:1). People of faith will work with many others in creating the future, searching in solidarity for creative and courageous ways to overcome suffering and its causes. People of faith will also bring their own particular motivation and vision, rooted in their religious beliefs. Ultimately, Christians will face suffering and political and economic challenges and will take action because they trust in God. This is not a pie-in-the-sky optimism but a profound conviction about the God revealed by Jesus.

"And what reason do I have to consider this abyss [of emptiness, despair, night, and death] as truer and more real than the abyss of God? It is easier to let oneself fall into one's own emptiness than into the abyss of the Blessed Mystery. But it is not more courageous or truer. This truth, of course, shines out only when it is also loved and accepted since it is the truth which makes us free and whose light consequently begins to shine only in the freedom which dares all to the very height. . . . [This truth] gives me the courage to believe in it and to call out to it when all the dark despairs and lifeless voids would swallow me up."[24] Karl Rahner's words capture the insight of the Christian tradition into trust. Even in the midst of systemic evils and staggering suffering from AIDS, nothing can snatch us out of God's hands.

Where does such trust come from? Christians find the source of this trust in Jesus's own experience and then in the community's experience of Jesus. Scripture scholars have helped us to appreciate that at the heart of Jesus's living and dying was a loving relationship with God and a bold, creative proclamation of God's Reign. Here we find the foundation of Jesus's own trust. According to the Scriptures Jesus addressed God as "Father" and even "*Abba*." Some scholars say that Jesus chose this word that small children used to address their fathers. *Abba* is best translated "Daddy"; it conveys a sense of childlike simplicity and familiarity.

Other Scripture scholars have recently offered the image of patron for understanding Jesus's use of *Father*. Appreciating the cultural world of the first century suggests this alternative interpretation, which implies a mature personal relationship with the one who empowers and distributes benefits, emphasizing trust, responsibility, and fidelity.[25]

Although offering different emphasis, these images are important for our consideration of Jesus's experience because they point to a very profound relationship between God and Jesus. How did it develop? We have no way of answering in detail, but we can assume that this bond developed gradually as Jesus lived life, heard the Hebrew Scriptures, asked himself about his own response to God, listened to John the Baptist, and began his own prophetic ministry, taking time to be alone and to pray. The God of Abraham and Sarah, Moses and Miriam, Isaiah and Jeremiah was Father to Jesus.

We catch another glimpse into Jesus's experience of God in the parables. One of the most helpful is Luke 15:11–32, often called the Parable of the Prodigal Son. This parable about the possibility of reconciliation is better described, however, as the Parable of the Forgiving Father. The details are familiar: The younger son demands his inheritance, leaves home, spends all the money and finally returns to his father's house, asking to be treated as a servant.

Notice the actions of the father: He allows his son freedom even to waste the inheritance; he watches for his return; he forgives the son without any bitterness, throwing a party to celebrate; he goes out to console the angry older brother. In this parable Jesus is telling us a lot about his own experience of God. *Abba* is both a dispenser of goods and benefits and a forgiving, gentle parent. Jesus evidently feels very close to this personal God, a God who reaches out to all, both those who wander away and those who stay at home, a God he can trust.

Similar insights come from Jesus's proclamation of the Reign of God, a central image in the Gospels. Simply put, the Reign means that God's power is at work in a particular situation. God's saving presence is found there. The Reign (also called Kingdom or Sovereignty or Empire) does not imply a particular place or time; the Reign is present whenever and wherever God's loving presence is manifested. The miracles of Jesus are symbols of God's Reign breaking into our world, of healing and salvation overcoming brokenness and sin (as we saw in chapter 2 with the leper).

Jesus used parables to speak about the Reign of God. Although he thus risked being misunderstood, Jesus allowed his listeners to make the connection between what he was talking about and what they were already expecting. He usually upset many of their preconceived notions of God's righteousness and power. Yet he took a chance that his words would touch the people in their depths and that they would act upon this discovery. He did so because he believed that the Reign of God, so evident in his own experience, could—and would—be recognized by others.

At times the Gospels begin Jesus's parables with the statement, "The Reign of God is like . . ." At other times, this statement is only implied. In Luke 8:4–15, for instance, Jesus simply begins, "A sower went out to sow his seed," and goes on to describe the different types of ground on which the seed fell. Part of *our* need in hearing this parable is to recognize that Jesus is describing very poor farming techniques. His hearers at the time, of course, knew that; they also knew that even the best techniques of the day produced about sevenfold. But in the parable the rich soil produces a hundredfold. Jesus is telling his listeners how surprising God's Reign is, how overflowing in goodness—not sevenfold but a hundredfold!

Because of Jesus's intimate relationship with God, Jesus experienced the presence of the Reign in and through his own life. And what he tried to tell others in his parables is that they could experience this Reign too![26]

Another section of the Gospels that provides rich insight into Jesus's experience of God's loving and saving presence is what we commonly know as the Sermon on the Mount (Matthew 5:1–7:29; in Luke's Gospel the location is level ground—see Luke 6:17–49). In these collections of Jesus's teachings we discover some of the surprise and goodness of the Reign: The hungry will be satisfied; those who weep now will laugh; those who are poor will be part of the Reign. The Sermon also gives other characteristics of life in the Reign: love of enemies, generosity, compassion, forgiveness, humility, and nonviolence. Luke's Jesus says, "Be merciful, just as your Father is merciful" (Luke 6:36). Matthew's Jesus says that God makes the sun "rise on the bad and the good, and causes rain to fall on the just and the unjust" (Matthew 5:45). At the center of Jesus's life was a deep trust in God.

This profound trust sustained Jesus even in his suffering and death. "Father, into your hands I commend my spirit" (Luke 23:46b). But his story did not end with the cross, with suffering and death. No, God raised Jesus to new and transformed life. The Resurrection can be understood as God's affirmation of Jesus's faithfulness and trust.

As faithful disciples, Jesus's followers attempted to embody and express this profound trust in God (although some, when they interpreted Jesus's death, slipped back into the ancient belief that violence saves—for more on this, see appendix I). The early communities did preserve and hand on Jesus's experience in light of their experience of the Resurrection, as evidenced in the Gospels quoted just above.

The Community of the Beloved Disciple, in particular, offers profound convictions about God as they reflect on the meaning of the Risen One in their midst. John's Gospel, written near the end of the first century, incorporated decades of preaching and reflection, of experiences of alienation from the Jewish community and acceptance in the Gentile community, of beginning dialogue with the philosophies of the age. The experience that began with personal encounter with Jesus of Nazareth leads to a vision reaching back to the beginning of time and offering a view of creation in and for Jesus. God's overflowing love is emphasized throughout the Gospel, beginning with the first verses.

"In the beginning was the Word, and the Word was with God, and the Word was God. . . . All things came into being through him, and without him not one thing came into being. . . . And the Word became flesh. . . ." The Prologue of John's Gospel (1:1–18) gives us this magnificent vision, proclaiming that all creation came to be in the Word, God's self-expression who became flesh, Jesus.

John's meditation of God's supreme act of love in the Incarnation (also see 3:16—"For God so loved the world that he gave his only Son, so that everybody who believes in him may not perish but may have eternal life") has led some theologians, as has been noted by Scripture scholar Raymond Brown,[27] to consider that this event alone was sufficient to save the world. Indeed, John's Gospel does not see Jesus's death as a ransom (unlike the Synoptic Gospels, for example Mark 10:45), nor does it use the language of sacrifice or atonement. There is instead emphasis on friendship, intimacy, mutuality, hospitality, service, and faithful love—revealing God's desire and gift for the full flourishing of humanity, or in other words, salvation (see the Farewell Address, John 13:1–17:26).[28]

Jesus's crucifixion (usually described as being "lifted up") is part of his "hour" of glorification, which also includes his resurrection and ascension. For John, this hour is not sacrifice but epiphany, the manifestation of God. If we pay attention to John's emphasis on the Incarnation and on the truth of God revealed in Jesus, we discover that what is at the heart of reality is a God who wants to share divine life. Surely we can trust this God of overflowing life and love.

Rahner's marvelous musings, then, about the dark abyss of suffering and the loving abyss of God have deep foundations. Trust in God is not some pie-in-the-sky piety, but a profound conviction rooted in the experience of the risen Jesus. Christians are an Easter people, trusting that good overcomes evil and that life overcomes death. Christians trust that God leads them in resisting evil and brings all to the fullness of life.

Indeed, belief in Jesus as the revealing Word leads to eternal life experienced now, that is, to participation in the very outpouring of divine life. This is another contribution of John's Gospel: Eternal life is not just life after death, but rather life in its fullness, life with and for God that Jesus reveals and that already begins when people through faith and love commit themselves to the kind and quality of life that Jesus embodies (see John 10:22–39, 11:1–45, 14:1–12).[29]

Christians still encounter the risen Jesus in word and sacrament, in service and suffering and silence, and in community and love. So Christians can help create the future by responding to the dark abyss of HIV and AIDS—to disease, death, and systemic evils—with lament, action, and profound trust in God. "HIV/AIDS brings with it new anguish and new terrors and anxiety, new trials of pain and endurance, new occasions for compassion. But it cannot change one enduring fact: God's love for us all."[30]

NOTES

1. See for example, Donald Senior, general editor, *The Catholic Study Bible* (New York: Oxford University Press, 1990), RG 241–RG 255.

2. Walter Wink, *Engaging the Powers* (Minneapolis: Fortress Press, 1992), 305.

3. Walter Brueggemann, "The Costly Loss of Lament," *Journal for the Study of the Old Testament*, vol. 36 (1986): 62.

4. Brueggemann, "Loss of Lament," 64.

5. Walter Brueggemann, *The Prophetic Imagination*, second edition (Minneapolis: Fortress Press, 2001), xii.

6. Brueggemann, *Imagination*, 56.

7. Brueggemann, *Imagination*, 65.

8. Brueggemann, *Imagination*, 65.

9. See especially Wink, *Engaging*.

10. Walter Wink, *The Powers That Be* (New York: Doubleday, 1998), 24.

11. Wink, *Engaging*, 9.

12. Wink, *Engaging*, 3.

13. Wink, *Powers That Be*, 4.

14. Wink, *Powers That Be*, 124.

15. Wink, *Powers That Be*, 63–111.

16. UNAIDS, *AIDS in Africa: Three Scenarios to 2025* (Geneva: UNAIDS, 2005), 4.

17. UNAIDS, *Three Scenarios*, 4.

18. UNAIDS, *Three Scenarios*, 13–15 and 50–59.

19. UNAIDS, *Three Scenarios*, 16; see also 102–37.

20. UNAIDS, *Three Scenarios*, 15; see also 60–101.

21. UNAIDS, *Three Scenarios*, 18; see also 138–75.

22. UNAIDS, *Three Scenarios*, 151–69.

23. UNAIDS, *Three Scenarios*, 12; what has been said here about Africa, of course, can apply to other areas as the pandemic continues to spread.

24. Karl Rahner, S.J., "Thoughts on the Possibility of Belief Today," in *Theological Investigations V* (Baltimore: Helicon Press, 1966), 8–9.

25. John H. Elliott, "Patronage and Clientism in Early Christian Society," *Forum*, vol. 3, no. 4 (December 1987): 39–48.

26. For this and other points in this section, see Arthur J. Dewey, "The Truth That Is In Jesus," *The Fourth R* (July–August 2003): 7–11.

27. Raymond E. Brown, *A Retreat with John the Evangelist* (Cincinnati: St. Anthony Messenger Press, 1998), 24.

28. See also Francis J. Molony, S.D.B., *The Gospel of John* (Collegeville: The Liturgical Press, 1998) and J. Massynberde Ford, *Redeemer: Friend and Mother* (Minneapolis: Fortress Press, 1997).

29. See the commentary on these passages in Arthur J. Dewey, *The Word in Time*, revised edition (New Berlin, Wis.: Liturgical Publications, 1990), 18–19, 29–31, 166–67.

30. National Conference of Catholic Bishops, *Called to Compassion and Responsibility* (Washington, D.C.: USCC Office of Publishing Services, 1990), 28.

Appendix I

The Mystery of God and Suffering

Suffering surrounds us. Mental and physical illness, poverty and starvation, wars and systemic violence of all kinds overwhelm individuals, communities, entire nations. People experience suffering in broken relationships and alienated families, in accidents and disease, in failed dreams and boring jobs, in dying and death. Many personal stories also include addictions, abuse, and other forms of violence. As we have seen throughout this book, the staggering suffering caused by HIV and AIDS is found in so many of these and other situations.

Such suffering often leads people to ask about God. "Who is God?" "How can a good and gracious God allow this to happen?" "Where is God in all this suffering?" "Is there a God?" Those directly involved in suffering often ask: "Why did this happen to me?" and sometimes even "What did I do wrong to be punished in this way?"

Humans have long searched for some satisfying insights into these and similar questions. The whole Book of Job in the Bible is dedicated to this topic. Christians have focused, in particular, on the suffering and death of Jesus in the hope of discovering meaning for suffering. Some of these biblical perspectives, however, fail to satisfy contemporary hearts and minds that long for the God of compassion revealed by Jesus.

In order to suggest a fitting response to our suffering, then, this appendix first considers the life and death of Jesus, including some of the dominant interpretations of his suffering and death. We will return to Scripture and Tradition for another perspective on Jesus's life and death, and see what this means both for our image of God and our response to suffering.

JESUS'S LIFE AND TEACHINGS

From the Gospels we learn three important points about Jesus and suffering: (1) Jesus resisted suffering and its personal and social causes and is frequently described healing persons; (2) Jesus rejected the conviction that suffering is the punishment for sin; (3) Jesus expressed a profound trust in a loving, compassionate, and present God.

First, many Gospel stories tell of Jesus healing the blind and sick. Matthew's Gospel summarizes this way: "Then Jesus went about all the cities and villages, teaching in their synagogues and proclaiming the good news of the kingdom, and curing every disease and every sickness" (9:35).

Second, deeply embedded in the Hebrew tradition is the conviction that suffering is punishment for sin, called the Law of Retribution. The people in exile in Babylon, for example, interpreted this political-social event as God's punishment for their failure to follow the covenant faithfully. This conviction appears in many religions and cultures. Jesus, however, rejected it. Matthew's Jesus in the Sermon on the Mount describes God as showering rain on evil persons as well as good ones (Mt 5:45). Similarly, John's Jesus heals the blind man and explicitly rejects the idea that suffering is punishment for sin (John 9:1–41, especially 2–5).

Third, implicitly and explicitly the Gospels reveal Jesus's intimate, loving relationship with God. Jesus' surprising use of *Abba* ("Daddy") to describe God conveys a sense of simplicity, familiarity, fidelity, and trust (as was described in chapter 8). The parables also give us a glimpse of Jesus' sense of God. The Prodigal Son (Luke 15:11–32) tells us a lot about the father, forgiving the son without any bitterness, celebrating his return, and consoling the angry older brother. *Abba* is a loving, forgiving, gentle parent. Even as he faced suffering and death, Jesus remained faithful to his call, always trusting God. In the resurrection, God confirms Jesus's faithfulness.

INTERPRETING A TERRIBLE DEATH

The life and teaching of Jesus highlighted the healing presence of a God of love and life. In the end, however, Jesus suffered a horrible execution. The mystery of suffering and death—first Jesus's and later others'—led the early Christian communities to search for light and meaning. They looked to their culture and their Hebrew Scriptures for possible interpretations. They included these insights in their preaching and eventually in the Christian Scriptures.

From culture they knew about ransom. From their Jewish practices they also experienced sacrifice and atonement. From their Wisdom literature they were familiar with the theme of the vindication of the Innocent Sufferer. From the prophet Isaiah (chapters 42, 49, 50, 52–53) Jesus's followers creatively used the songs of the Suffering Servant to interpret Jesus's suffering and death. The Messiah, of course, was not expected to be a suffering messiah. The facts of crucifixion and death jarred Jesus's followers into searching the Hebrew Scriptures for insight for proclaiming and interpreting his death (see the letter to the Hebrews, for example).

Scholars tell us that what the Bible understands by terms such as sacrifice and atonement may be quite different from the understandings that many of us have. For example, for Hebrew people, the blood of the sacrificed animal symbolized the life of the person or community. Pouring the blood on the altar was a symbolic gesture reuniting life with God. The sacrifices were an expression of the people's desire for reconciliation and union with God.

It must be noted, however, that even while emphasizing these more positive meanings of sacrifice, most of the scholars pass over in silence the fact that the ritual still includes violence and the death of the victim—dimensions that are foreign to Jesus's vision of the reign of God.

Throughout the centuries Christians have reflected on and developed these different interpretations, leading to a variety of theologies and popular pieties, some of them quite distant from the Scriptures and even farther from the vision of Jesus.

In the fourth century, St. Augustine spoke of satisfaction for sin in legal terms of debts and justice. A key development took place in the twelfth century when the theologian St. Anselm used St. Augustine's ideas to describe atonement for sin. Anselm, reflecting the medieval culture of his day, understood sin to be something like a peasant insulting a king. Reconciliation would require satisfaction for this insult to the king's honor. Sin, however, is an infinite offense against God that demands adequate atonement. While humanity was obliged to atone, no human could pay this infinite debt. Only God could do so adequately.

According to this twelfth-century view, that is exactly what Jesus, the God-Man, accomplished by his suffering and death. It was actually later theologians and preachers who added to Anselm's position by emphasizing blood and pain as the satisfaction that placated God's anger. Most Christians still grow up with such an understanding, although some are uneasy with this view, even if they do not know why.

This image of God—angry, demanding, even bloodthirsty—often appears in sermons, songs, and popular pieties today, although the focus is usually placed on Jesus's willingness to bear the suffering. Initially, this willingness to suffer for us may seem profoundly moving and consoling. But we must ask several questions of this interpretation. What does this say about God the Father? What kind of God could demand such torture of the beloved Son? Is this the God revealed by Jesus in his words and deeds?

JESUS IS NOT PLAN B

There is an alternative interpretation of the life and death of Jesus, also expressed in the Scriptures and throughout the tradition. This view, perhaps only on the margins of many people's religious understanding and devotion, is completely orthodox. Indeed, it offers perspectives much closer to Jesus's own experience and vision.

What, briefly, is the heart of this alternative interpretation? It holds that the whole purpose of creation is for the Incarnation, God's sharing of life and love in a unique and definitive way. God becoming human is not an afterthought, an event to make up for original sin and human sinfulness. Incarnation is God's first thought, the original design for all creation. The purpose of Jesus's life is the fulfillment of the whole creative process, of God's eternal longing to become human. Theologians call this the primacy of the Incarnation.

For many of us who have lived a lifetime with the atonement view, it may be hard at first to hear this alternative, Incarnational view. Yet it may offer some wonderful surprises for our relationship with God. God is not an angry or vindictive God, demanding the suffering and death of Jesus as payment for past sin. God is, instead, a gracious God, sharing divine life and love in creation and in the Incarnation. Such a view can dramatically change our image of God, our approach to suffering, our day-to-day prayer. This approach is rooted solidly in John's Gospel and in the letters to the Colossians and the Ephesians.

Throughout the centuries great Christian theologians have contributed to this positive perspective on God and Jesus. From the Cappadocian Fathers in the fourth century (St. Basil, St. Gregory of Nyssa, St. Gregory of Nazianzus) to Franciscan John Duns Scotus in the thirteenth century to Jesuits Teilhard de Chardin and Karl Rahner in the twentieth century, God's gracious love and the primacy of the Incarnation have been proclaimed.

In the late twentieth century, theologian Catherine LaCugna pulled together many of these themes in her book *God for Us.* She uses and expands the Cappadocians' wonderful image of the Trinity as divine dance to include all persons. Borrowing themes of intimacy and communion from John's Gospel and Ephesians, she affirms that humanity has been made a partner in the divine dance not through humanity's own merit but through God's election from all eternity. She writes: "The God who does not need nor care for the creature, or who is immune to our suffering, does not exist. . . . The God who keeps a ledger of our sins and failings, the divine policeman, does not exist. These are all false gods. . . . What we believe about God must match what is revealed of God in Scripture: God watches over the widow and the poor, God makes the rains fall on just and unjust alike, God welcomes the stranger and embraces the enemy."[1]

Theologian Edward Schillebeeckx, O.P., has also questioned the traditional interpretation of Jesus's death. In Part Four of his book *Christ*, Schillebeeckx strongly affirms and holds together God's goodness with suffering, both in Jesus's life and in all humans' experience. Schillebeeckx does not try to explain away the reality of suffering and evil in human history, but sees them as rooted in finitude and freedom. Still he stresses that God's mercy is greater, as seen in Jesus's ministry and teaching. God does not want people to suffer but wills to overcome suffering wherever it occurs.

Such a God could not require the death of Jesus. Schillebeeckx states: "*Negativity* cannot have a cause or a motive in God. But in that case we cannot look for a divine *reason* for the death of Jesus either. Therefore, first of all, we have to say that we are not redeemed *thanks* to the death of Jesus but *despite* it."[2] Schillebeeckx adds, "Nor will the Christian blasphemously claim that God himself required the death of Jesus as compensation for what *we* make of our history."[3]

The emphasis on Jesus as God's first thought can free us from violent images of God and allows us to focus on God's overflowing love. This love is the very life of the Trinity and spills over into creation, Incarnation, and the promise of fulfillment of all creation. What a difference this makes for our relationship with God! Life and love, not suffering and death, become the core of our spirituality and morality.

THE ABYSS OF SUFFERING

But what about the "dark abyss" (Psalm 88) of suffering? The Incarnational approach with its emphasis on God's overflowing love leads us beyond our natural question of "Why?" and suggests three elements of a response to suffering: (1) acknowledge the suffering and then lament, (2) act, and (3) trust in God (as explained and exemplified in chapter 8).

Again, briefly, the first step in responding to suffering is simply being truthful, avoiding denial (which could be so easy) and admitting the pain and horror of the suffering, whatever the cause. We must never glorify suffering. Yes, it can lead us to deeper maturity and wisdom, but suffering can also crush the human spirit. Following the lead of the Psalmist, we can express our pain in lament. Such crying out allows us both to grieve and to grow into a mature covenant partner with God.

Awareness of suffering and relationship with God allow and inspire our action, the second element in our response to suffering. We acknowledge that at times our choices have caused personal and social suffering, so one form of action is moving toward repentance and a change of heart. We also suffer from sickness, including HIV and AIDS, and many other personal challenges. In this suffering we need to reach out to others, to ask for help, to receive what they offer, to allow them to accompany us in the dark abyss. As we reach out to other humans, so too we move toward God (who may seem very distant) in lament, service, praise, or gratitude.

Following the life and ministry of Jesus, we work as individuals and as communities to overcome and end suffering. Our deeds include remaining with others in their suffering, along with action concerning political and economic issues. The needs are so great and the systemic issues so complex—what can one person do? We can search in solidarity with others for creative and courageous ways to overcome suffering and its causes in our world, as suggested in the earlier chapters. We cannot do everything, but we can at least do one thing. The third element in our response to suffering, trust in God, is of course especially challenging in the dark times of suffering. Our usual response is initially just the opposite. We question how God could cause this suffering or at least allow it. We ask why. We may complain to God or even begin to doubt God's existence. That is exactly why the lament psalms can be so helpful, matching our experience and emotions. The lament allows us to stay in conversation with God, gradually moving to a new trust.

Jesus, of course, is a marvelous example of trust in God. His deep, trusting relationship with *Abba* grounded his life and teaching. "Are not two sparrows sold for a penny? Yet not one of them will fall to the ground apart from your Father. And even the hairs of your head are all counted. So do not be afraid; you are of more value than many sparrows" (Mt 10:29–31).

Lament and action and trust, however, do not remove the question of suffering. Suffering remains a mystery, not a problem to be solved. We stand with Job at the end of his bold contest with God: "What can I answer you? I put my hand over my mouth" (40:4).

THE LOVING ABYSS OF GOD

The emphasis on creation-for-Incarnation, culminating in the resurrection, gives us great hope as we confront the overwhelming suffering of HIV and AIDS. God does not desire suffering but works to overcome it. God did not demand Jesus's suffering and does not want ours. In the context of trusting this gentle God, we lament and act to overcome suffering, even as we acknowledge its incomprehensibility and marvel at God's remarkable respect of human freedom. We know that some suffering results from persons' evil choices (war, injustice, oppression). We know that other suffering simply happens in a world that is not yet fulfilled (earthquakes, debilitating diseases). Suffering, however, is not fully understandable. So, we move past "Why?" to ask instead: "How can I respond? What can we do now?" A profound trust in a compassionate God allows us to ask these questions and then to act, with surprising peace and hope.

Finally, the mystery of God and suffering invites us to prayerful meditation. A suggestion: recall Michelangelo's magnificent sculpture
Pieta. The grieving mother of Jesus holds his dead body in her arms.
Feel the pain, the sorrow, the horror. Then allow the sculpture to become a symbol, to take on even greater meanings. First, perhaps, the
symbol of the world's mothers holding their dead sons and daughters,
ravaged by AIDS. Then let the sculpture speak of a gentle God holding
God's sick and dying world. Finally, let it be God holding your broken
spirit.

Our God suffers with us, to use human terms. In the depths of suffering we too may cry out: "My God, my God, why have you forsaken
me?" In the darkness, we may need to express our lament, even defi-
ance, but finally our trust that the gracious, gentle God holds our sick
and broken bodies and spirits. How could it be otherwise for the God of
life and love, the covenanted partner, the tender and gracious parent?

We can trust because there is more: our God is a God of resurrection,
of new life. Jesus's story did not end with suffering and death, but with
new and transformed life. And Christians are an Easter people. That
truth, ultimately, is at the very heart of our response to suffering. God
suffers with us, leads us as individuals and as community in resisting
evil, and brings us all to the fullness of life.

NOTES

1. Catherine Mowry LaCugna, *God for Us* (New York: HarperSanFrancisco,
1991), 397.

2. Edward Schillebeeckx, *Christ* (New York: Seabury Press, 1980), 729.

3. Schillebeeckx, *Christ*, 728.

Appendix II

Preparing Now for the Hour of Death

As we wrestle with end-of-life issues, is there anything else we can do NOW? Yes! We can fill out an *advance directive*, that is, a form giving our wishes concerning future health care.

One type of advance directive is a *living will*. This form is a statement prepared in advance so that people, while competent, can direct their families and physicians concerning the type of treatment they want or do not want if they become terminally ill and are no longer able to express their desires about medical treatment.

The living will, because it is filled out in advance, can never foresee all the details of a future illness and the related medical procedures. That is its major limitation. On the other hand, it gives evidence of reflection and desires concerning what kind of treatment the person wants.

A second type of advance directive is the *health care power of attorney* (also called "health care surrogate" or "proxy" but different from the usual "power of attorney"). In this document an individual gives another person the legal authority to make health-care decisions when the individual is no longer able to do so. The decisions made by the appointed person are based on the current medical condition of the patient and on the patient's previously expressed desires concerning treatment. As a result, this form of dealing with dying-and-death situations seems to be preferable. It does not rely merely on a previously written statement to cover all possible situations.

A lawyer or physician can provide the proper form. A copy of the advance directive ought to be given to the appointed person, to one's physician, and to a family member. Besides creating a legal document, the process is just as important for the communication (with the appointed person, the physician, and family) that is a necessary part. The time for this discussion and appointing is NOW—and not at a time of crisis. Also, this process is necessary for all of us, whatever our age; it is not just for senior citizens.

All this may seem like too much effort. It is not! The whole process of planning now for the hour of death is a concrete way to express care and love for family and friends since they will be the ones faced with the difficult and painful decisions. It is a way to relieve fears of prolonged dying by being attached needlessly to machines. It is a way to counteract the movement toward euthanasia. It is a way to express concern for the appropriate use of the earth's limited resources.

Because many people do not appreciate the richness and nuance of the Catholic tradition on end-of-life issues and because many put off the simple procedures of filling out an advance directive, parish ministers provide a great service to people by gathering large and small groups to discuss the tradition and to walk through sample directives. Such conversation and planning can have sober moments but also be a prayerful experience, acknowledging the final mystery of life and expressing trust in our gracious God.

Selected Bibliography

Administrative Board of the United States Catholic Conference. *The Many Faces of AIDS: A Gospel Response*. Washington, D.C.: USCC Office of Publishing Services, 1987.

———. "Political Responsibility." *Origins*, vol. 25, no. 22 (16 November 1995).

Administrative Committee of the U.S. Conference of Catholic Bishops. "Faithful Citizenship." *Origins,* vol. 33, no. 20 (23 October 2003).

Angell, M.D., Marcia. "Euthanasia." *New England Journal of Medicine*, 319, no. 20 (17 November 1988).

Beauchamp, Tom, and James Childress. *Principles of Biomedical Ethics*. 4th ed. New York: Oxford University Press, 1994.

Bernardin, Joseph Cardinal. *Consistent Ethic of Life*. Kansas City: Sheed & Ward, 1988.

———. *A Moral Vision for America*. Washington, D.C.: Georgetown University Press, 1998.

Bonneau, Normand, Barbara Bozak, Andre Guindon, and Richard Hardy. *AIDS and Faith*. Ottawa: Novalis, 1993.

Borg, Marcus J. *Meeting Jesus Again for the First Time*. New York: Harper Collins Publishers, 1994.

Brown, Raymond E., *A Retreat with John the Evangelist*. Cincinnati: St. Anthony Messenger Press, 1998.

Brown, S.S., Raymond, Joseph Fitzmeyer, S.J., and Roland Murphy, O.Carm., eds. *The New Jerome Biblical Commentary*. Englewood Cliffs: Prentice Hall, 1990.

Brueggemann, Walter. "The Costly Loss of Lament." *Journal for the Study of the Old Testament*, vol. 36 (1986).

———. *The Prophetic Imagination*. 2nd ed. Minneapolis: Fortress Press, 2001.

Butwell, Ann, Kathy Ogle, and Scott Wright, eds. *We Make the Road by Walking: Central America, Mexico, and the Caribbean in the New Millennium.* Washington, D.C.: EPICA, 1998.

Cavanaugh, John, et al. *Alternatives to Economic Globalization: A Better World Is Possible.* San Francisco: Berrett-Koehler, 2002.

Cimperman, Maria. *When God's People Have HIV/AIDS.* Maryknoll, N.Y.: Orbis Books, 2005.

Clements, Mark, et al. "Modeling Trends in HIV Incidence among Homosexual Men in Australia." *Journal of Acquired Immune Deficiency Syndromes*, vol. 35, issue 4 (1 April 2004).

Congregation for the Doctrine of the Faith. *Declaration on Euthanasia.* Washington, D.C.: USCC Office of Publishing Services, 1980.

Connors, Jr., Russell B., and Patrick T. McCormick. *Character, Choices, & Community: The Three Faces of Christian Ethics.* Mahwah, N.J.: Paulist Press, 1998.

Crossin, John W. *What Are They Saying about Virtue?* Mahwah, N.J.: Paulist Press, 1985.

Czerny, S.J., Michael. "University and Globalization: Yes, But." *Santa Clara Lectures*, vol. 9, no. 1 (7 November 2002).

Dewey, Arthur J. "The Truth That Is In Jesus." *The Fourth R* (July–August 2003).

———. *The Word in Time.* rev. ed. New Berlin, Wis.: Liturgical Publications, 1990.

Drane, James F., and John L. Coulehan. "The Concept of Futility: Patients Do Not Have a Right to Demand Medically Useless Treatment." *Health Progress*, 74, no. 10 (December 1993).

Editors. "Signs of the Times." *America,* vol. 190, no. 3 (2 February 2004).

Elliott, John H. "Patronage and Clientism in Early Christian Society." *Forum*, vol. 3, no. 4 (December 1987).

Esack, Farid. *HIV, AIDS & Islam.* Observatory, South Africa: Positive Muslims, 2004.

Fairchild, Amy L., James Colgrove, and Ronald Bayer. "The Myth of Exceptionalism." *Journal of Law, Medicine & Ethics*, vol. 31, no. 4 (Winter 2003).

Flannery, O.P., Austin, ed. *Vatican Council II.* Northport, N.Y.: Costello Publishing Company, 1996.

Ford, J. Massynberde. *Redeemer: Friend and Mother.* Minneapolis: Fortress Press, 1997.

Forman, Walter B., ed. *Hospice and Palliative Care.* Sudbury, Mass.: Jones and Bartlett, 2003.

Gaylin, M.D., Willard, Leon R. Kass, M.D., Edmund D. Pellegrino, M.D., and Mark Siegler, M.D. "Doctors Must Not Kill." *Journal of the American Medical Association,* 259, no. 14 (8 April 1988).

Glanton, Dahleen. "Emerging Face of HIV." *Chicago Tribune*, 28 March 2004.

Green, Edward C. "The New AIDS Fight: A Plan as Simple as ABC." *New York Times*, 1 March 2003.

Gremillion, Joseph, ed. *The Gospel of Peace and Justice*. Maryknoll, N.Y.: Orbis Books, 1976.

Guinan, Michael D. *To Be Human before God: Insights from Biblical Spirituality*. Collegeville: The Liturgical Press, 1994.

Gula, S.S., Richard M. *Reason Informed by Faith: Foundations of Catholic Morality*. Mahwah, N.J.: Paulist Press, 1989.

Gustafson, James M. *Protestant and Roman Catholic Ethics: Prospects for Rapprochement*. Chicago: The University of Chicago Press, 1978.

Halperin, Daniel T., et al. "The Time Has Come for Common Ground on Preventing Sexual Transmission of HIV." *Lancet*, no. 364 (27 November 2004).

Hamel, Ronald, and Michael Panicola. "Must We Preserve Life?" *America*, vol. 190, no. 14 (19–26 April 2004).

Holy See. *Catechism of the Catholic Church*. Liguori, Mo.: Liguori Publications, 1994.

Irwin, Alexander, Joyce Millen, and Dorothy Fallows. *Global AIDS: Myths and Facts*. Cambridge, Mass.: South End Press, 2003.

Jaffe, Carolyn, and Carol H. Ehrlich. *All Kinds of Love*. Amityville, N.Y.: Baywood Publishers, 1997.

John Paul II. "The AIDS Epidemic." *Origins*, vol. 20, no. 15 (20 September 1990).

———. "A Church Responding to the Sick and the Poor." *Origins*, vol. 20, no. 15 (20 September 1990).

———. *The Gospel of Life*. Boston: Pauline Books and Media, 1995.

———. "Is Liberal Capitalism the Only Path?" *Origins*, vol. 20, no. 2 (24 May 1990).

———. *On Social Concern*. Washington, D.C.: USCC Office of Publishing Services, 1987.

Kammer, S.J., Fred. *Doing Faithjustice*. Mahwah, N.J.: Paulist Press, 1991.

Kass, M.D., Leon R. "Neither for Love nor Money: Why Doctors Must Not Kill." *The Public Interest*, vol. 94 (Winter 1989).

Kavanaugh, John F. "Artificial Feeding." *America*, vol. 190, no. 20 (21–28 June 2004).

———. *(Still) Following Christ in a Consumer Society*. Maryknoll: Orbis Books, 1991.

Keenan, S.J., James F. ed. *Catholic Ethicists on HIV/AIDS Prevention*. New York: Continuum, 2002.

Kelly, Kevin T. *New Directions in Sexual Ethics: Moral Theology and the Challenge of AIDS*. London: G. Champman, 1998.

Kim, Jim Yong, Joyce Millen, Alec Irwin, and John Gershman, eds. *Dying for Growth: Global Inequality and the Health of the Poor*. Monroe, Me: Common Courage, 2000.

LaCugna, Catherine Mowry. *God for Us*. New York: HarperSanFrancisco, 1991.

Mann, Jonathan, Daniel J. M. Tarantola, and Thomas W. Netter, eds. *AIDS in the World*. Cambridge, Mass.: Harvard University Press, 1992.

Massaro, S.J., Thomas. "Judging the Juggernaut: Toward an Ethical Evaluation of Globalization." *Blueprint for Social Justice*, vol. LVI, no. 1 (September 2002).

McCormick, S.J., Richard A. *Corrective Vision: Explorations in Moral Theology*. Kansas City: Sheed and Ward, 1994.

———. "'Moral Considerations' Ill Considered." *America*, vol. 166, no. 9 (14 March 1992).

———. *Notes on Moral Theology 1965 through 1980*. Washington, D.C.: University Press of America, 1981.

———. *Notes on Moral Theology 1981 through 1984*. Lanham, Md.: University Press of America, 1984.

———. "*Vive la Difference!* Killing and Allowing to Die." *America*, vol. 177, no. 18 (6 December 1997).

McGowan, J., et al. "Risk Behavior for Transmission of Human Immunodeficiency Virus (HIV) among HIV-seropositive Individuals in an Urban Setting." *Clinical Infectious Diseases*, vol. 38, no. 1 (1 January 2004).

McNeil, Jr., Donald G. "Plan to Battle AIDS Worldwide Is Falling Short." *New York Times*, 28 March 2004.

Messer, Donald E. *Breaking the Conspiracy of Silence*. Minneapolis: Fortress Press, 2004.

Miller, Cari L., et al. "The Future Face of Coinfection." *Journal of Acquired Immune Deficiency Syndromes*, vol. 36, Issue 2 (1 June 2004).

Molony, S.D.B, Francis J. *The Gospel of John*. Collegeville: The Liturgical Press, 1998.

National Conference of Catholic Bishops. *Called to Compassion and Responsibility: A Response to the HIV/AIDS Crisis*. Washington, D.C.: USCC Office of Publishing Services, 1989.

———. *Economic Justice for All*. Washington, D.C.: USCC Office of Publishing Services, 1986.

———. *The Harvest of Justice Is Sown in Peace*. Washington, D.C.: USCCB Publishing, 1994.

Novak, Michael. *The Catholic Ethic and the Spirit of Capitalism*. New York: Free Press, 1993.

O'Brien, S.J., Kevin, and Peter Clark, S.J. "Drug Companies and AIDS in Africa." *America*, vol. 187, no. 17 (25 November 2002).

O'Connell, Timothy E. *Principles for a Catholic Morality*. rev. ed. New York: HarperCollins, 1990.

O'Donovan, Leo J., ed. *A World of Grace*. New York: The Crossroad Publishing Company, 1987.

Ohio Catholic Conference of Bishops. *Hopes and Fears: Pastoral Reflections on Death.* Columbus: Catholic Conference of Ohio, 1993.

Overberg, S.J., Kenneth R., ed. *AIDS, Ethics & Religion.* Maryknoll, N.Y.: Orbis Books, 1994.

———. *Conscience in Conflict.* 3rd ed. Cincinnati: St. Anthony Messenger Press, 2006.

———. *Into the Abyss of Suffering.* Cincinnati: St. Anthony Messenger Press, 2003.

———, ed. *Mercy or Murder?* Kansas City: Sheed & Ward, 1993.

Paris, S.J., John. "Active Euthanasia." *Theological Studies,* 53, no. 1 (March 1992).

———. "Hugh Finn's 'Right to Die.' " *America,* vol. 179, no. 13 (31 October 1998).

Paris, John, and Richard McCormick. "The Catholic Tradition on the Use of Nutrition and Fluids." *America,* vol. 156, no. 17 (2 May 1987).

Paterson, Gillian. *Women in the Time of AIDS.* Maryknoll, N.Y.: Orbis Books, 1996.

Paul VI. *Evangelization in the Modern World.* Washington, D.C.: USCC Office of Publishing Services, 1976.

Porco, Travis, et al. "Decline in HIV Infectivity Following the Introduction of Highly Active Antiretroviral Therapy." *AIDS,* vol. 18, issue 1 (2 January 2004).

Post, Stephen G. "Adolescents in a Time of AIDS." *America,* vol. 167, no. 11 (October 17, 1992).

Rahner, S.J., Karl. *Theological Investigations.* Vol. II. Baltimore: Helicon Press, 1963.

———. *Theological Investigations.* Vol. V. Baltimore: Helicon Press, 1966.

Schillebeeckx, Edward. *Christ.* New York: Seabury Press, 1980.

Senior, Donald, gen. ed. *The Catholic Study Bible.* New York: Oxford University Press, 1990.

Shannon, Thomas. *Bioethics.* 3rd ed. Mahwah, N.J.: Paulist Press, 1987.

Sheldon, Kathleen, ed. *Courtyards, Markets, City Streets: Urban Women in Africa.* Boulder, Colo.: Westview Press, 1996.

Shelton, James, Daniel Halperin, Vinand Nantulya, Malcolm Potts, Helene Gayle, and King Holmes. "Partner Reduction Is Crucial for Balanced 'ABC' Approach to HIV Prevention." *British Medical Journal,* no. 328 (10 April 2004).

Singer, M.D., Peter A., and Mark Siegler, M.D. "Euthanasia—A Critique." *New England Journal of Medicine,* 322, no. 26 (28 June 1990).

Smith, Ann, and Enda McDonagh. *The Reality of HIV/AIDS.* Maynooth, Ireland: Trocaire, Veritas, CAFOD, 2003.

UNAIDS. *AIDS in Africa: Three Scenarios to 2025.* Geneva: UNAIDS, 2005.

Urbina, Antonio, and Kristina Jones. "Crystal Methamphetamine, Its Analogues, and HIV Infection: Medical and Psychiatric Aspects of a New Epidemic." *Clinical Infectious Diseases*, vol. 38, no. 6 (15 March 2004).

USCCB Committee on Pro-Life Activities. *Nutrition and Hydration: Moral and Pastoral Reflections.* Washington, D.C.: USCCB Publications Service, 1992.

Veatch, Robert M., and Carol Mason Spicer. "Futile Care: Physicians Should Not Be Allowed to Refuse to Treat." *Health Progress*, 74, no. 10 (December 1993).

Wanzer, M.D., Sidney H., Daniel D. Federman, M.D., S. James Adelstein, M.D., Christine K. Cassel, M.D., Edwin H. Cassem, M.D., Ronald E. Cranford, M.D., Edward W. Hook, M.D., et al. "The Physician's Responsibility Toward Hopelessly Ill Patients: A Second Look." *New England Journal of Medicine*, 320, no. 13 (30 March 1989).

Wink, Walter. *Engaging the Powers.* Minneapolis: Fortress Press, 1992.

———. *The Powers That Be.* New York: Doubleday, 1998.

Wohl, Amy Rock, et al. "Recent Increase in High-Risk Sexual Behaviors among Sexually Active Men Who Have Sex with Men Living with AIDS in Los Angeles County." *Journal of Acquired Immune Deficiency Syndromes*, vol. 35, issue 2 (1 February 2004).

Index

About the Author

Kenneth R. Overberg, a Jesuit priest, is professor of theology at Xavier University in Cincinnati. He received a Ph.D. in social ethics from the University of Southern California. Among his books and articles are six national award-winners, including *Conscience in Conflict*, now in its third edition from St. Anthony Messenger Press.